— EVERYDAY —
MIRACLE MAKER

— EVERYDAY —
MIRACLE MAKER

*7 self-transformation keys to unlock
your miracle-making mindset*

SILVANA LA PEGNA

Creator: La Pegna, Silvana, author.
Title: Everyday Miracle Maker: 7 self-transformation keys to unlock your miracle-making mindset / Silvana La Pegna.

ISBN: 9780648011514 (hardback)

ISBN: 9780648011507 (paperback)

ISBN: 9780648011521 (ebook)

Subjects: Spiritual healing. Self-care, health mind and body. Holistic medicine. Miracles.

Publisher
Sacred Light Pty Ltd
PO Box 1293
Double Bay NSW 1360

Cover and text design: Natasha Solley and Josie Fox.
Cover photographs by: Helen Coetzee © Silvana La Pegna
Styling and Hair: Robbie Sylva
Make-up Artist: Leah Drapper
Publishing Consultants: Pickawoowoo Publishing Group
Printing: Lightning Source (US/UK/AUST)

The author does not provide medical advice or prescribe the use of any technique as a form of treatment for physical, emotional or medical problems without the advice of a physician. The intent of the author is only to offer information to help you in your quest for spiritual and emotional wellbeing. In the event you use any of the information in this book for yourself, the author and the publisher assume no responsibility.

CONTENTS

INTRODUCTION

The Everyday Miracle Maker examples presented in this book are composites of several similar stories. None represents an identifiable individual. Sexes have been switched frequently and pseudo names created. Similarly, circumstances, locations and events were changed to protect an individual's identity. Any similarity to any real person's name or identity is coincidental.

INTRODUCTION

You may have experienced miracles in the past as mysterious spontaneous events; this book is about how you can *consciously* create miracles in your life. Everyday.

As a coach and mentor I have spent my entire career learning, applying and benefiting from principles to help my clients transform their lives into ones that are more productive and joyous. I've discovered there are 7 self-transformation keys that when combined with daily practices can help us to invite everyday miracles into our lives.

We live in a conscious universe. Everything is made up of energy vibrating at different frequencies. What you believe, think, say and do sends invisible signals through your body and to everyone and everything around you.

This book will teach you how to broadcast and receive the right signals, messages, opportunities and desires for you. It'll teach you how to improve the quality of your life by understanding how you can positively influence your mind, body and environment.

Your feelings and energy levels are inextricably connected. When you're low in energy, you can feel awful. When you have loads of energy, you can feel great. If you're lost, scattered, unfulfilled, or just want more out of life, learning how to become an Everyday Miracle Maker can be... life-changing for you.

Everyday miracles can't be forced. They're acts of deliberate co-creation that allow you to attract what you want with less stress. It's about having the right tools. I'll show you how to get there; all you need to do is stay committed and focused to reaching new heights. I'll teach you how to draw in immediate opportunities and experiences to convince yourself that your mind (or consciousness) has an organising power that extends far beyond your physical body. Many of the principles shared in *Everyday Miracle Maker* once transcended scientific explanation for the effects they produce are now gradually being understood through consciousness studies and advances in neuroscience.

Sometimes we overlook our own intuitive flashes and impulses because we have a fixed rational idea of what is right and proper for us to pursue. Other times we overlook the signs because we want our choices to be acceptable to our partners, family, friends or peers. We think we'll feel better with their validation, but in reality we need to fully accept what we want for ourselves.

I've learnt that to succeed and be fulfilled by your successes you have to put as much emphasis on developing your *inner* world as you put into developing your *outer* world. Being overly reflective and focusing mainly on your inner world (or primarily on your outer world) sets up an imbalance that affects and distorts your perception of your life.

Miracles are awe-inspiring because they interrupt the natural processes and improve them in a way that we didn't anticipate. We connect with stories of a person meeting their soul mate and miraculous healings because they give us hope and remind us that there exists an unseen power that can affect someone, or something, to intervene in our life when we need it most.

This book is the culmination of three decades of research, personal experience and knowledge. You may not have recognised synchronicities, acts of grace, lucky breaks, windfalls or being at the right place at exactly the right moment as everyday miracles, but there is no doubt in my mind; when a spontaneous blessing of any size arrives when you need it – it's an everyday miracle.

Perhaps you're attracted to this book by your intuition, whether you're consciously aware of it or not. If you're open to the idea, you'll identify know-how, insights and reminders that will jump out at you from the pages. Pay closer attention and take notes so you don't forget what resonates with you.

When I work with clients I have a sensory response. When I pay attention to their voice, body or name, I see intuitive flashes of people, places, events and things connected to them while being impressed by their mental and emotional state. It's as if an illuminated path shows me how to connect the pieces of their story.

After many years of emotional turmoil, professional confusion and physical trauma I discovered a new path, one that relied on developing my intuition to receive astonishing insights and wisdom. And that changed my life, literally. I spent the next eight years observing, studying and working with my clients, family, friends and on myself with frequency-shifting approaches.

Our bodies are a dynamic energy system. When working as a Medical Intuitive, I used my intuition to detect frequencies of disharmony in human energy fields. To do this I attuned myself to my clients' energy field and explained to them how they could do the same to identify and shift frequencies in their bodies to improve their physical, mental or emotional wellbeing.

I observed that many mental and emotional conditions that clients complained about were visible in their energy bodies – the fields that emanate from our subtle energy bodies (the counterpart of the physical body) told me everything I needed to know. Knowing how to translate the information in these fields gives us access to another level of our reality. What we think and feel persistently has a real and direct effect on our subtle energy bodies; over time those effects become visible in the health of our physical body and life. When our beliefs and thoughts are unsupportive, we can feel depleted of energy and over time we can become unwell. When we choose support-ive beliefs and thoughts, we cultivate wellness. Energetically, this creates vibrational harmony and coherence throughout our body. Conversely, unsupportive beliefs and thoughts create disharmony and incoherence, which can lead to illness. This realisation moved me from working as a Medical Intuitive to a coach and mentor. From what I'd learnt through observing and working with the energy fields of my clients, I felt drawn to sharing my insights and experiences to promote high-level wellbeing which I believe can be significantly assisted by reveal-ing and experiencing our soul's desires.

I've coached hundreds (probably thousands) of clients resulting in thousands (or hundreds of thousands) of every-day miracles for them, from small windfalls, fortuitous career transitions, exceptional business opportunities to healings and accomplishing soul's desires.

This book is dedicated to the Everyday Miracle Makers of the past, present and future. Every time a person chooses to embrace my 7 self-transformation keys to switch on their miracle-making mindset, they're inviting everyday miracles into their life.

Chapter One

BELIEFS HAVE FREQUENCIES

BELIEFS HAVE FREQUENCIES

Your entire body is a broadcasting and receiving tower. The vibrational frequencies of your beliefs can immediately affect your wellbeing because your mind is not confined to your head.

Like radio waves, these vibrational frequencies are invisible to the human eye. They're like arrows shooting and pulsing through the air looking for targets that resonate with them.

Have you noticed how certain people stay in your life for a while, whereas others just come and go like visitors? Often when we transform or drastically change our beliefs around something it can have a profound knock-on effect to the overall energetic signature of who we are. It can repel or attract people, places, events and things into or away from our life. Energy doesn't discriminate with finger-pointing; it doesn't say that you're good and they're bad. It just matches up like-minded things and sets unlike-minded things apart.

Have you ever spent time with someone that left you feeling drained and flat, or energised? Often people we resonate with vibrationally boost our energy, while people we *don't* resonate with can leave us feeling lacklustre.

Energy increases and decreases can also be affected by your thinking. Any healthy practice that increases your self-awareness will assist you to recognise the quality of your thinking. From my experience, there are two factors that have the most significant effect on your energy levels: What your mind focuses on; and how you choose to respond to it. By increasing your self-awareness you can become better at choosing supportive beliefs and thoughts over unsupportive ones. The meaning you place on anything that happens in your life and how you choose to interpret it can help you to maintain your energy levels and experience positive emotions, as long as you choose to see it as either supportive or neutral.

Vibrational Frequencies of food and water

Food and water emit vibrations with specific frequencies.

Nutrient-rich foods that are organic or pesticide-free have vibrational frequencies that are more harmonious, healthy and helpful for our bodies. Water that is free of toxic contaminants is the same.

If you feel flat and low in energy, think about what you are consuming from an energetic point of view. What you *choose* to consume most of the time is what matters because you are absorbing its vibrational frequencies. Choose foods free of chemical additives and try to stay away from highly processed, genetically altered or mistreated food. It'll help you maintain healthier vibrational frequencies in your body.

Blessing a meal before you eat it is a ritual in many cultures. It's a simple way to focus your energy to increase the vibrational frequency of the food. And it's easy. Just give thanks to the food and where it came from while holding an intention of how you'd like it to serve your body, mind, energy and overall wellbeing. You can either do this mentally, or out loud, whichever works best for you.

I bless food (raise the vibrational frequency) as I am preparing it. Recently a close friend's elderly mother was in intensive care in hospital. The treatment she was undergoing had left her body depleted of energy; she was extremely ill and had lost a significant amount of weight. I offered to make a week's supply of my healing chicken soup in the hope it would help restore her. As I made the soup I thought about my friend and her mum and blessed it with the restorative qualities of healing and love. I pictured her mum sitting up in bed, loving my soup and getting stronger. Two weeks later I received news that her mum had refused *all* food except my soup and told her daughter, "I don't know what's in this soup but it's making me feel a lot better, I know it". Her acute condition eased and within a month she returned home.

Vibrational Frequencies of music and art

Just as food and water emit vibrational frequencies that can be supportive to you, so too can music and art. The next time you're listening to a piece of music or looking at a piece of art notice how it makes you feel. Compile a playlist of music and songs on your phone that instantly uplift your mood when you listen to them. Listen to this playlist anytime you're finding it challenging to stay upbeat and optimistic. I'm an advocate for using any tool that helps me maintain the optimal vibrational frequencies to remain aligned to my soul's desire. While writing *Everyday Miracle Maker* I compiled a playlist of music that I enjoyed daily. This music was pivotal in helping me maintain alignment.

For me, the vibrational frequencies I enjoy from looking at art are just as powerful as listening to my music playlists. I choose art for my home that elicits emotions and memories that I enjoy connecting with, after all I'm soaking up these vibrational frequencies everyday!

Everyday Miracle Maker Exercise: Your beliefs have frequencies

Try this to convince yourself that your beliefs have frequencies that can immediately affect your wellbeing.

Place one hand over your heart centre and say out loud *believing* these words are true: I'm hopeless; no one wants to be in my company. Pay attention to the frequency feeling in your body. It should feel bad.

Using the same process, place one hand over your heart again, but this time say: I'm amazing, kind, generous, warm and successful, and people are drawn to me. Pay attention to the frequency feeling in your body. It should feel good. Again, pay attention to your energy levels. Can you feel the increase in your energy overall? As the frequency of your thoughts increases to a higher level of awareness, so does the feeling of having an increase in your energy level. These are always linked.

The change is the frequency contrast of those two beliefs. Your body gives you immediate feedback through how you feel. The words you use most of the time tell your body what energetic diet you *prefer* to consume. Everyday Miracle Makers are committed to a high vibrational frequency diet.

The vibrational frequency of your intentions and the language you choose to use carries a subtle and powerful energy. All day and night your body is receiving and broadcasting vibrational frequencies. It's sending and receiving signals that affect you and your environment. Learning to pay attention to the changing feelings and sensations in your body can help hone your intuition and decode these signals. A feeling may bring flashes of insight that can give you a sense of whether something is good (or bad) for you, depending on whether you feel an increase or decrease in your energy levels.

Your beliefs affect the quality of the water in your body. This is important to keep top of mind when you consider our bodies are made up of approximately 70 per cent water. Energy doesn't judge positive from negative; it lines you up with your most dominant vibrational frequencies. You choose the quality of energy you broadcast into the world by renewing and committing every day by choosing your beliefs, thoughts, actions and language that support the life you want. Being an Everyday Miracle Maker is about deliberately *choosing* to manage the quality of the energy you broadcast through your body into the world.

New York Times best-selling author and researcher Dr. Masaru Emoto believes that water responds to subtle invisible energy from humans. His book *Hidden Messages* explores the theory that intentions and language focused directly into a bottle of water can result in beautiful (or ugly) water crystals (seen through microscopes and high-speed photography). Scientist Dr. Hans Jenny spent years researching the effect of sound waves on water. He determined that the higher the frequency, the more beautiful and intricate the pattern.

The quality of the subtle energy you broadcast from your mind and body can be positive or negative. The choice is yours.

When you speak, the vibrational frequency of the words you've chosen instantly affects you and your environment. What you say broadcasts energy into your future. Positive words are energetically strengthening, while negative words are energetically draining and can generate internal stress and confusion. It's like an alarm going off and the security doors to the logic and reasoning rooms shutting down. And no one can function effectively when there's an alarm ringing.

Everyone talks to himself or herself; we *all* talk to ourselves in our head. You might know this as your inner dialogue, self-talk or mental chatter. Your language carries powerful vibrational frequencies, whether those words are internalised, or vocalised. Speaking in ways that support what you envision for yourself is critical in staying congruent to your soul's desire. The infinite consciousness that co-creates with you to make everyday miracles happen, works faster and more powerfully when you are congruent. You need to walk your talk and talk your walk towards what your soul desires.

Pay attention to how you talk about pursuing your soul's desire to friends, your partner, family or colleagues. The most supportive language you can use matches your self-talk; it needs to stay upbeat, *positive* and optimistic.

If you share what you are doing with others and it's met with negativity or scepticism, you won't be affected.

The Everyday Miracle Maker understands that the words they choose shape the quality and tone of their inner dialogue so they keep their language positive.

You Have a Force Field

You have an energy field that extends beyond your physical body which is like a force field. Your body, including your organs, is connected to and surrounded by other energy fields. Just like a magnet, these fields exist both within and around our organs and body. These energy fields have the ability to attract or repel the energy fields of other people, places and things around you.

So far science has identified many types of energy fields. It's likely you've heard of the terms magnetic, electric and gravitational fields yet many more exist invisibly (and powerfully).

Your energy body's ability to send and receive vibrational frequencies is not a new discovery; it's been observed, researched and practised for thousands of years by many sacred traditions and cultures around the world from Australia to India.

Frequency Shifting Tool

I'm often asked to assist in frequency shifting and intention setting for clients in their homes and offices, and before shoots and events.

For over a decade I've been doing this with *Sacred Light Aromatherapeutic Mist*. It's a combination of 7 key essential oils that have been blessed to increase and raise the vibrational frequency of your inner and outer space. Essential oils have healing and supportive frequencies, so if you struggle to get into the right headspace for creative work, meditation or decision-making, you'll find it useful. It's also wonderful to clear the air of any unsupportive energy at home or work. If you need a positivity boost (whether it's related to work, family or your romantic life) then set an intention in the room with *Sacred Light Aromatherapeutic Mist*. It'll help you create supportive frequency shifts in your mind, body and in the spaces you occupy.

→ *Learn more about Sacred Light Aromatherapeutic Mist at everydaymiraclemaker.com*

Chapter Two

MINERS, MOUNTAINEERS AND PILOTS

MINERS, MOUNTAINEERS AND PILOTS

The Everyday Miracle Maker needs to be flexible; your inner and outer environments go through cycles of change, just like the weather does each season.

There are three main perspectives to be mindful of: Maybe, you've needed to withdraw for some inner reflection (miner); or perhaps you've needed a challenge (mountaineer); or maybe you've needed to remove yourself from the minutiae of your life to obtain a zoomed-out higher perspective (pilot).

Miners work underground; most of the time they aren't seen. Their bodies expend a lot of effort, energy and force to compensate for tough working conditions. But the payoff can be gold and diamonds.

Mountaineers climb up and down peaks searching for a higher perspective. The reward comes from reaching the summit and seeing something that few people experience first-hand. But at some point you have to come down the mountain.

Then there's the Pilot, who has a bird's eye view of the sky, mountains and ground. They navigate their way with a powerful engine, but at some point the plane needs to land and refuel.

We can go through our life as just a miner, just a mountaineer or just a pilot and not realise we are missing out on the benefits the other perspectives can offer us.

It's valuable to recognise that we need to allow ourselves to experience *all* perspectives to engage in our lives in a healthy and productive way. Not too much inner reflection, not too much challenge and not so out of reach that we lose touch with the reality of our lives and the quality of our relationships with those around us.

The Everyday Miracle Maker embraces all perspectives, understanding that at some point she or he will find themselves as the Miner, the Mountaineer or the Pilot (and experience their respective environments). What's important is to stay fluid and not get stuck in any one perspective.

Do the quiz to find out which perspective type is most dominant for you. Visit everydaymiraclemaker.com

Chapter Three

MIRACLE-MAKING CHALLENGES

MIRACLE-MAKING CHALLENGES

Everything around you has the ability to drain your energy levels, whether you realise it or not.

Communication Drains

Advances in technology have made it easier and faster for us to communicate than ever before, but the opportunity cost is high. We're expected to be contactable 24/7 and respond immediately to emails, texts and phone calls. Most people are wading through around 10 personal and subscription emails, plus up to 30 work emails each day. If you're feeling overwhelmed by the pressure to respond, cut yourself some slack; you aren't alone.

Tip: Turn off notifications and sound on your email and phone to reduce distractions. Respond to communications only at set times throughout the day.

Information Drains

We're constantly accessing information whether it's through our phones, laptops, tablets or even our watches – we're rarely unplugged.

When Google started in September 1998 users were submitting around 10,000 searches per day. Within a year that figure jumped to 3.5 million a day. In 2016, there were 3.5 billion searches a *day* www.internetlivestats.com/google-search-statistics/. But does access to more information than we've ever had before mean we're advantaged?

Tip: Switch off computers, TV and other technology at least 30 minutes before bedtime to help improve your sleep.

Productivity Drains

Because we have the tools to work faster, we are. We're squeezing more into our day than ever, and because our downtime is more valuable, we have to be selective about how we spend it. Too much work and we start building resentment; it's easy to forget the joy of doing what we love. The converse is also true though; if we have too much free time, complacency and procrastination set in.

Tip: When working on a task and it feels like a drain, pause and look for a couple of advantages for yourself in what you are doing to reset your mindset.

Competition Drains

We've been conditioned to believe competition is necessary for success through conventional learning, communities, corporations *and* in our relationships. If you don't compete to win (or if you choose *not* to compete) you're not taken seriously and you're voted off the island. The anxiety of competing can result in exhaustion on many levels – mental, physical, emotional and spiritual.

Tip: Choose to improve your personal best in what you do rather than comparing yourself to others, it's healthier and more helpful in the long term.

Self-Confidence Drains

When we have low self-confidence in several dimensions of our lives, we can rely heavily on external validation and recognition. When we believe what others think about us is more valuable than what *we* think of ourselves we are susceptible to self-confidence drains.

Self-confidence is an inner feeling that is developed through skills and competencies, persistence and repetition. It isn't something we magically feel without dedicating considerable time, energy and effort towards. For instance, you can't expect to feel self-confident in cooking if you rarely cook new dishes or try new techniques. Entertaining unsupportive thoughts about yourself when you haven't made a commitment to the area you want increased self-confidence in, only diminishes any self-confidence you wish to develop.

Tip: To increase your self-confidence in a specific area you need to increase your skills, knowledge and experience in it.

Self-Talk Drains

Driving everything you think, feel, do and say is your unconscious belief system. It operates like computer software; it encodes how you engage with your body, your life and the world around you (whether you're aware of it or not).

Some of your unconscious beliefs might support you in achieving your soul's desire, but others may be counter-productive to it, and you might be unaware of how these beliefs are sabotaging your efforts at success. The quality of your beliefs determines the quality of your thoughts. Worry, fear and negative thinking generate stress in your body that immediately drains your energy. Your brain on stress is like a clenched first. When you're experiencing high levels of stress, your ability to access the parts of your brain that can help you restore calm becomes difficult.

Some sabotaging beliefs are chameleons; they're harder to identify and transform on your own. But with professional support most unsupportive beliefs can be isolated and upgraded to help you succeed where you desire it most.

You may have many unsupportive beliefs impacting on your choices. It could be a belief created in early childhood. Some beliefs act like a rogue safety program that tries to protect you from a threat (sometimes imagined) that influences your behaviour without you realising it. It can influence you to turn down new experiences under the guise of self-preservation, but it's actually creating obstacles and blocks between you and what you want.

Tip: When you aren't thinking kindly and supportively about yourself or others, disrupt that self-talk by upgrading your beliefs and thoughts with a U-turn and go in the opposite direction.

Overwhelm Drains

When we allow ourselves to think that we can't manage a situation because it seems too complex or challenging we can enter the slippery domain of overwhelm drains. The longer we remain overwhelmed the more anxiety we can feel. At some point the Everyday Miracle Maker may feel overwhelmed. However, you do have the ability to manage the degree of overwhelm you experience, and move through it. One of the most effective approaches in my experience is to keep your body relaxed, acknowledge what you are feeling, then bring your entire awareness into the present-moment and focus on managing one task at a time to completion. Being fully present in the environment you're physically in (keeping your mind and body tethered together) counteracts feelings of anxiety.

You can minimise the impact that disappointments have on you. Whether you didn't get the job you were hoping for, a business deal fell through, a relationship ended or you didn't get the exam results you wanted, you can choose your response. When you decide to approach challenges like opportunities, you immediately move energy towards more supportive frequencies. By keeping your thoughts neutral if something doesn't go your way rather than allowing them to become pessimistic, you can access creative solutions to navigate challenges more effectively. When you're stressed you can't easily problem-solve which contributes to feeling more stressed out.

Tip: *Reorient your mind back to your body's location in the present moment in whatever you're doing and then tell yourself aloud and with conviction "I can do this".*

Chapter Four

MIRACLE RECALL

MIRACLE RECALL

An important part of being an Everyday Miracle Maker is to recall the everyday miracles that have occurred in the past. It's important to remind your conscious and unconscious mind that everyday miracles are familiar to you. Recall keeps the energy of those miraculous happenings close. When they remain within your field of attention, it makes it easier for you to identify new everyday miracles and maintains the vibrational resonance that assists in creating more of them.

When I started working as a Medical Intuitive, I'd taken a significant drop in my income. I'd moved from a corporate career to pursuing what my soul desired, and as I was in the early stages, money was tight. Around that time, I was asked to volunteer my services to a spiritual development and healing group that met two evenings per week at a location 45 minutes away from my home. Though I was concerned about the cost of petrol in travelling there, I went ahead with it because my intuition was encouraging me. The day after I agreed, I was in a department store paying for my purchase, when my eyes were drawn to a competition on the counter to win $250 in petrol vouchers. I felt a strong nudge from my intuition to enter the competition.

A week later I received a call from the department store advising me I was the winner. My intuitive impulse was my soul encouraging me towards this opportunity for further growth.

When we surrender to our soul's guidance we are always taken care of. That day I remember looking up into the sky from the department store car park and saying, "Universe, you amaze me, thank you".

Everyday miracles can find their way to you through people, places, television, the computer, your phone, results, winnings, overcoming fears, doing something new or unfamiliar, saying yes and remaining optimistic about your life (when it is easier to say no and stay in your comfort zone).

Last year when finalising a business proposal for a client, I had a nagging feeling I was being conservative with my recommendations; I didn't think their budget would allow me to implement a comprehensive solution based on a discussion we'd had previously. I took a walk before sending the proposal to my client and asked my intuition for validation around the proposal's constraints. Within 5 minutes my awareness was drawn to a pink envelope on the footpath with two large words on it: THINK BIG. I felt 100 per cent certain in every cell in my body that it was a sign; that was my answer. I ran to my office, added the extra recommendations in my proposal and pressed send on my email. Within two hours I received a call from my client to say they loved my proposal and accordingly increased the project budget.

Be on the lookout for signs that are leading you to everyday miracles; they can turn up in the most unusual places.

Everyday Miracle Maker Exercise: Identify everyday miracles

Using your intuition glance over the following list and circle 3 types of everyday miracles that you're drawn to. Then take a moment to recall and make notes of the specific details that you experienced. By doing this exercise you'll be reminded of the spontaneous everyday miracles that have already occurred for you. By becoming an Everyday Miracle Maker you'll learn principles and practices that can allow you to create them more often.

- Synchronicities
- Aha moments
- Acts of grace
- Being inspired with solutions
- A chance meeting
- In the right place at the right time
- Being inspired with a brilliant idea or invention
- Serendipity
- Coincidence
- A soul mate connection
- The impossible becomes possible
- Experiencing a spontaneous healing
- Winning against high odds
- A financial windfall
- Receiving a blessing

- Divine intervention
- Good fortune
- Witnessing an uplifting phenomena
- Communication from a loved one in spirit.
- Receiving a gift of what you need just when you need it.
- A Godsend

If you've experienced other types of everyday miracles add them to this list.

Chapter Five

7 KEYS TO BECOMING AN EVERYDAY MIRACLE MAKER

7 KEYS TO BECOMING AN EVERYDAY MIRACLE MAKER

I have identified after decades of observation, research and study that there are 7 keys to unlocking your miracle-making mindset.

Key #1: Soul

We are souls. Our soul's mission in having a human life is to gain wisdom through experiences. Our soul-self can choose to pursue experiences in life that enable us to learn, grow and evolve to reflect more of our spiritual essence of *love*.

Key #2: Authenticity

Authenticity is honouring our feelings and expressing the truth of who we know ourselves to be and what's right for us. It's our soul's unique form of self-expression and our power-place.

Key #3: Intuition

It's the voice of our soul that's available to us 24/7. Our heart and gut are sensitive gauges of intuitive guidance, and can offer us vibrational feedback on opportunities, people, places, events and things. The sensations and responses that vibrational feed-back evokes in our minds and bodies (whether it feels good or bad) is information we can use to decide whether to move towards or away from anything (or anyone).

Key #4: Gratitude

Gratitude is an amplifying frequency that is heart centred. Offering gratitude is recognition that goodness has and is showing up in our life, and we have things to be thankful for now.

Key #5: Alignment

Alignment is being in agreement. When our beliefs, thoughts, actions and language reinforce each other, we're aligned. This produces a feeling of certainty that we're on the right path and that all our energy is travelling in the same direction.

Key #6: Creativity

Creativity is the act of creating something we've imagined. It's an action that has value; not just something we think about (and never do). Expressing our creativity can heal our mind, body and soul.

Key #7: Optimism

Optimism is believing in ourselves and our ability to move through and manage any adversity, trusting it's all going to work out because we deserve goodness in our lives.

The soul's greatest desires are love and wisdom.

Chapter Six

KEY 1: SOUL

KEY 1: SOUL

You are a soul. Your soul is the energy of your consciousness. Your soul-self can choose to pursue experiences in life that enable you to learn, grow and evolve.

I use several terms when discussing the highest universal intelligence imaginable. It might be the Universe, Infinite Consciousness, God, Great Spirit, the Creator, Source, Creative Intelligence – they all have the same meaning for me. Use the term that resonates with your outlook on life.

The soul's mission in having a human life is to gain wisdom through its experiences, and its driver (and spiritual essence) is love.

The soul is the immortal part of us that is outside of time and lives on after our physical bodies die. Because the soul is connected to the human body, it is affected by our life experiences.

Having worked with energetic and spiritual healing for many years, I learned that our soul requires healing to support the healing of our minds and bodies.

The greater our soul's wisdom, the greater our understanding and appreciation of how intricately connected we are to all life. One of the ways our unconscious connection to other people has been shown is through thousands of studies worldwide that provide evidence for the existence of telepathy, particularly with people we are emotionally connected to. The illusion of separateness from one another and the world around us is perpetuated by the ego and this is the cause of most misunderstandings, pain and suffering.

Our soul evolves through our intentions and choices, including our environment, for the better or worse. Yet the soul is also continuously influenced by the purity of our spirit to keep evolving. As a soul we get to decide how we wish to navigate this life; either through fear or with an increasing capacity for love. When our desires change from being exclusively self-serving to making time to be of service to others, studies show it can make us happier and healthier.

Because our soul-self has more insight and influence from our spirit than our personality, its guidance is wiser and more valuable. The degree we allow our soul-self to guide our decisions determines the quality of our life experiences.

How the soul's whispers can guide you

Listen out for the many ways your soul-self tries to guide you in helping you navigate your life decisions. By listening you'll discover new knowledge and skills to assist you moving towards what you want. Like most people you'll be used to giving most of your attention to your analytical mind. Your soul speaks through intuition – it's not the mental chatter of an anxious mind, so you need to learn to listen in a different way.

Some of my clients' most common intuitive messages have included:

- Focus on restoring wellbeing

- Recommit to a relationship – whether it's personal, romantic or familial
- Start a business to reveal more of your abilities
- Return to school as a mature student
- Learn a foreign language to make new global connections
- Be open to meeting your soul mate
- Practise forgiveness to surrender any form of payback
- Increase your financial wealth without compromising your integrity
- Improve work/life balance
- Explore after-life research after losing a loved one
- Let go of anger
- Avoid gossiping
- Re-engage in your social life after break-up or loss
- Be more accepting of yourself and loved ones
- Love your body unconditionally
- Stop relying on other people to take care of your financial future
- Develop your intuition
- Practise greater patience in your relationships
- Reinforce positive habits
- Slow down and quit worrying you're not doing enough
- Stop blaming others or yourself
- Practise generosity
- Redirect your attention from being the problem solver in your children's and partner's lives, to your life

- Accept people as they are by letting go of the need to change them
- Take 100 per cent responsibility for every dimension of your life

Your soul will have many desires that you can pursue, but the one you now feel a persistent call to is the one that's worth exploring. Soul's desires have a personal and spiritual development imperative that isn't always immediately understood or appreciated. Everything in life contains meaning, but some things will mean more to you than others. Your soul's desires can be hidden within what's *most* meaningful to you in your life.

When you start revealing your soul's desires, you'll automatically trigger your imagination and then your creativity to assist the conscious planning process required to solve any problems to accomplish it.

If you're not experiencing what you want to be, do or have, it means you are out of alignment with what you desire. When you practise being an Everyday Miracle Maker you'll know how to create alignment to restore harmony to your life by shifting the frequencies of what you believe, think, say and do to be more optimal in order to accomplish what your soul desires. Refer to my BTAL Alignment Process™ on page 194 for further assistance.

What's suppressed is expressed

I grew up in a large Italian family that focused on socialising with food. The lead-up to important events like Christmas and

Easter were hectic with food preparations for our immediate and extended family and friends, but it was an exciting time; the anticipation of laughter, lots of lovingly hand-made food, growing deeper bonds with relatives and dancing and singing to Italian songs were something we all looked forward to.

But it wasn't just holidays when our house buzzed with family and food; my mum loved to cook and bake so our house was a social hub for relatives.

Every Sunday afternoon my aunties and cousins would come over to chat and eat my mother's freshly baked sponge cake with homemade vanilla custard. I was fascinated by these visits, not just because there was cake, but because of the conversations that happened between the adults. I was engrossed by news of family members' difficulties, issues and challenges – even though I was a child. I was curious about the human condition. Eventually I became a sounding board for colleagues, friends and strangers who were all drawn to confide in me, trusting that I would; a) treat their concerns and troubles with sensitivity; and b) show them how to find the answers within to their problems.

What these conversations taught me was that we're responsible for most of our unhappiness. I always believed that our souls spoke to us through our intuition; I don't recall anyone ever telling me, it was just something I knew as a child.

Our soul is always trying to direct us, but most of the time we aren't listening. But the challenge was that back then, few people I knew understood or believed in intuition, let alone grasped the concept of soul's guidance. As my intuitive impulses from the world around me increased, so too did the feeling of being overwhelmed. Instead of embracing and supporting my unfolding intuitive ability, I suppressed it, not because I thought it wasn't valuable, but because I wanted to fit in, be accepted and validated by friends, family and colleagues.

Gradually my body suffered from a mental disconnect from my soul's guidance. Everyone I associated with complained about their life and so did I. I assumed that whinging was normal – just a side effect of life. I was conditioned to believe that life wasn't meant to be easy. Every time my unhappiness peaked to new levels of misery, it had a peculiar knock-on effect. I'd lose my patience, quit my job, have weird accidents or get sick. And I don't mean any kind of ordinary sick; I'd get a terrible cold or flu that would last for weeks, or a nasty and mysterious bug that doctors found difficult to diagnose.

And then I got *visibly* sick. I was diagnosed with Guttate Psoriasis – a condition that riddled my entire body with red scaly teardrops. My skin was literally crying. My unhappiness had rendered me pessimistic and blind to the opportunities and possibilities around me. I was out of sync with my soul's guidance. While I couldn't see that it was a blessing at the time (and that wallowing in self-pity and blame was one of the causes) it course-corrected me mentally and emotionally back to my soul-self and towards my soul's desire.

I was covered with sores, suffering from depression, unable to work, in terrible mental pain, itchy 24/7 and at the end of my rope. Despite seeing many doctors, I wasn't getting significantly better. It wasn't until I visited a holistic medical centre in Sydney that I began to find relief.

Martine Negro – an acupuncturist, energetic healer and lecturer who worked at the centre – helped me arrive at the insight that suppressing my intuition was getting in the way of healing my condition. Within 12 weeks of her treatment plan most of my symptoms had disappeared.

A light switched on in my head.

Instantly, I could see my unsupportive actions that, up until that point were invisible to me. I'd been reading books on spiritual development subjects since I was 15 years old, and while on a conscious level I agreed with most of the principles in them, my unconscious mind wasn't having a bar of it. Because my beliefs weren't congruent with my thoughts, actions and language, there was little change in my life.

Discovering that my beliefs influenced my actions *freed* me. Upgrading my beliefs to be supportive created a lighter, brighter atmosphere around me. This new atmosphere allowed me to act in ways that attracted the opportunities I wanted.

Intuition

Intuition is a form of creative higher intelligence. Repressing it was causing a build-up of energy within me that was fighting to be expressed. It was like a pressure cooker with the valve closed and the only way it could escape was through my skin.

The healing process set me on a completely different career path. When I realised the immense value of the healing and self-transformational work I was doing, I was compelled to use my new knowledge to help others. I wanted to share the short-cuts I'd learned. Soon I was working at the same holistic medical centre in Sydney supporting others to transform their own challenges.

Sometimes tuning in to the whispers of your soul's desire can be challenging. But if you take steps to deliberately listen to it, you can identify what needs upgrading in your life.

Your parents may have wanted you to follow in their foot-steps professionally. Perhaps you settled down and had children because it was expected of you. Or maybe you were taken from your path by religious beliefs, partners' opinions, financial commitments and other societal pressures. If you allow the opinions of others to direct your life, or their judgements to affect what you think you should or shouldn't be doing, you won't be able to hear your soul's whispers trying to guide your decision-making.

Putting yourself first (even if it's not what your loved ones want for you) doesn't mean you're being disrespectful. It means you are choosing to follow what feels right for you. Taking full responsibility for your life direction also means accepting the consequences of your choices. It can take time to rid yourself of people-pleasing behaviour but, if you don't put yourself first, who will?

Your soul's voice isn't necessarily a chorus of angelic voices and celestial trumpets; often the whispers can call out to you through pain and hurt. Areas of your life that produce feelings of agony, frustration, sadness and anger are telling you something. When you give any area of your life your full attention and hold a genuine desire to improve it, your soul will activate your intuition and the guidance will follow.

If you blame others for any perceived misfortune or feeling, you're stuck facing the wrong direction; and have your back to your soul's guidance. Turn around. The moment you surrender resentments you'll feel the intensity and power of your soul's healing light up your heart and life.

Your intuition can also nudge you to take action towards making a positive difference in achieving your soul's desire. If you struggle with any of the following, and you are getting a persistent inner impulse to address these, it's your soul using your intuition to give you a heads-up.

- Keeping your word
- Following through with projects
- Finishing what you start
- Speaking the truth (kindly)
- Dropping the façade and being real (and owning it)
- Being authentic to yourself, no matter what people think of you

Too often we fall into the trap of referencing ourselves by the shallow wants of our ego, but that's just a harbinger of anxiety and emptiness. Getting hooked on it means we experience feelings of incompleteness.

When we get in touch with our soul's desire we start to:

- Feel more enthusiastic (it may not have happened for years)
- Commit to future events (when we usually resist them)
- See opportunities (instead of seeing problems)
- Say yes (rather than saying no)

Identifying and exploring your soul's desires will cause an uplifting frequency shift in your mind and body that can be felt.

EDUCATE YOUR EGO

Think of your personality as having two parts. One part is informed and aware, and the second part is uninformed and unaware. The unaware part is the ego. It serves to help you survive, but it can overshoot its purpose. The ego has a bad habit of distorting reality and generating memories that are unhelpful and unsupportive.

When you find yourself ruminating on stressful and imaginative stories in your head your nervous system responds to the intensity of what you are thinking because your mind doesn't know the difference between what is real and what's imagined. This is true for your positive and supportive imaginings as it is for your negative ones. When you react to circumstances in your life like you're in a life or death situation when you aren't, that's the level of internal stress your mind and body will experience. When your thoughts extend beyond self-preservation and survival you evoke and encourage your soul-self to guide you.

There is another beneficial reason for acknowledging that we co-create with a higher power. Whether you recognise it to be your soul-self, or infinite intelligence, acknowledging this power helps keep your ego in check. When you're open to the understanding that a higher spiritual reality exists beyond the limitations of physical life, your soul can keep drawing your attention to the myriad ways you're connected to the world around you. When you put your life in context to a broader perspective it can have the effect of making you less consumed with just securing your needs and wants and also motivates you to assisting others secure what they need.

The degree to which you allow your soul to guide your decision-making makes all the difference to the quality of life you experience. Have you ever wanted to be, do or have something badly, but when you got to be, do, or own it you weren't content? The ego is a master at conning you into believing that having that thing (or experience) will bring long-lasting happiness. Because the ego is unaware and doesn't know any better, it *believes* its decision-making is in your best interests, but largely it's a calculating little fox focused on pleasure and self-preservation.

Decision-making that is guided by the soul instead of the ego is gentle, kind and satisfying. It's a conscious choice between harmony over disharmony; inclusiveness over exclusiveness, and love over fear. Celebrating achievements driven by the ego can fade quickly, leaving you underwhelmed and searching for another accomplishment; you're on the hunt for more self-gratification.

So, how do you know what you wish to pursue is driven by your ego or your soul? At times this can be difficult to know with absolute certainty. However, rest assured your soul has the power and ability to *influence* your decision-making. It does this by inspiring you through your intuition to make a *course-correction* to support your self-development if you are heading in the wrong direction. As your level of self-awareness increases you become more subtly aware of whether you are in alignment with your soul's desire or not.

See your soul-self as your wisdom keeper. It sends you intuitive impulses to the likely consequences of your decisions and inspires you with alternatives when your decisions could take you off your path. It'll give you feelings of reassurance and certainty when you're on track. Learn to listen inwardly for your soul's guidance. When you listen to its persistent whispers, you turn up the clarity of the guidance. As you practise becoming an Everyday Miracle Maker by applying the 7 self-transformation keys in your life with greater degrees of success, your overall vibrational frequency will increase, and as it does you'll find it easier to communicate with your soul-self.

What your soul desires is personal to you; no one can possibly know with more certainty than you what your soul needs to experience. When you respond to the whispers of your soul, your life takes on a deeper meaning, which will bring you a more enduring level of contentment. Keep focused on evoking your soul's guidance whenever you need it, don't save asking for special occasions. Ask and expect an answer.

As a kid I was a ballroom dancer. I'll always remember the feeling of dancing in a championship and feeling the tap on the shoulder to leave the dance floor from one of the roaming adjudicators. The idea was they narrowed down the dancers often leaving three couples dancing for first, second and third place. Whenever we felt an adjudicator was walking towards us we'd occasionally sneakily try to avoid their hand making contact with either of us. But when it did occur, my partner Andrew and I would walk off the floor and watch the remainder of the competition from the sidelines. When your soul wants you to course-correct, it can feel like a tap on the shoulder. What I don't recommend is you ignore it and push on regardless. *The smart thing to do is hit pause, move to the sidelines and take time out to review your plans. Sometimes you're meant to make adjustments and get back on the floor and sometimes it's just not the dance your soul wants you in.*

LISTEN TO THE WHISPERS

If you're regularly unmotivated or bored it can be a sign that you need to connect to yourself at a deeper level and lean into experiences that allow you to grow and develop.

Everyone's soul speaks to them. But not everyone wants (or is ready) to hear what it's saying, or calling them towards. Have you heard your soul calling out to get your attention, but you chose to turn towards distractions instead? This can happen when you convince yourself that your lack of contentment is caused by your external environment; something you want added or removed from it.

When unconsciously you believe you're lacking something significant in yourself or life you may look for distractions. This could manifest itself in the following ways:

- Working more than necessary
- Spending hours on social media particularly when you wake-up or before bed
- Drinking heavily
- Needing to be entertained constantly
- Serial dating
- Always needing to be in a relationship
- Gambling regularly
- Drug taking to be social
- Giving advice to people who haven't asked for your opinion

- Dwelling on negative self-talk without taking action to turn those words around

- Binge eating

- Shopping constantly

Permanent relief comes from turning your attention towards your inner world, to get closer to your soul's whispers. Exploring this can free you from the discomfort you might be experiencing.

If you **can't** hear your soul whispering there's always a reason. You might be:

- Stuck in survival mode
- Be struggling financially
- Challenged to think positively about your life
- Comparing yourself to others
- Criticising yourself
- Knee-deep in depression
- Fearful you won't like what your soul wants you to know

Social media can give you the impression other people's lives are happier and more exciting or peaceful than yours. Keep in mind there will always be people who choose to show you what they want you to see (which could be far from the reality of their life). Comparisons are a waste of precious energy. No matter how well you know a person, all your conclusions about their life are largely just your perception.

Whether you're affected by distraction or not, embrace the *Everyday Miracle Maker* mindset and you'll take your attention and energy to a higher level.

I dropped out of high school early because I found conventional learning challenging. I was dyslexic but had no idea I was. In those days I wasn't identified as having a brain that was wired differently. Instead I was branded lazy and easily distracted, but in reality I often put in double the work of my classmates just to keep up. This led me to becoming disruptive and I struggled at school. It wasn't a place of happy memories.

I always regretted not finishing high school – in spite of my stuggles, I loved learning. So I returned to learning as a mature age student and sat the university entrance exam several times hoping to gain admission to earn a degree.

I knew I'd have to face and transform every learning obstacle that had overwhelmed me in the past, but this time I was better prepared. It was important for me to move through the adversity rather than turn back, so giving up was not an option.

It wasn't easy.

The first time I sat the university entrance exam I failed. I was disappointed, but determined to try again.

The second time I sat the exam I failed. Even though I was disheartened, I wasn't devastated. It didn't send me into a downward spiral of self-loathing like failing tests or exams had done at school; I recognised that something within me had changed. Instead of it infecting my self-esteem like it had before, I felt calm and optimistic. This frequency shift allowed me to regroup, refocus and try again.

On my third attempt, I passed. I was ecstatic. I danced and sang all through my apartment like I'd won 1st prize in the lottery. In a way, I had.

My "win" was life transforming. I'd been able to do something I never thought possible. Standing on the stage in a cap and gown at my graduation ceremony at the age of 32 was one of the proudest moments in my life. My soul's desire of having a Bachelor's Degree had finally been brought to life after years of living in my imagination.

Your soul-self is your truest self.

EVERYDAY MIRACLE MAKER EXAMPLE – SOUL

Name: Hannah

Age: 25

Hannah was angry with her family. She'd been seething for years.

She'd been raised in a family that couldn't understand her passion for community and social work, insisting she get a job and focus on earning an income.

I spent time listening to her and explained that the areas in our life that give us the most pain (or joy) are often where our path forward can lie. As her family's opinions caused her the most pain, Hannah believed that her soul's desire could only be fulfilled by pursuing an opportunity that was the antithesis of what her family wanted for her.

I shared a process with her, which I called *toggling up to soul and down to personality.* If you've ever had multiple applications open on your computer desktop you'll know the function of toggling between applications.

I asked Hannah to view her family from her soul's point of view; without judgement and with unconditional love. Then, toggle back to her personality (which the ego is connected to) and pay attention to the contrast of her feelings and insights. Upon reflection Hannah recognised her true soul's desire was to experience a loving relationship with her family by having an open mind and heart towards them – people she'd never seen as needing assistance because they were financially affluent.

Hannah began addressing her perception of her family's disregard for the less fortunate. Her soul's guidance led her to understanding that she needed to accept her family for who they were; and whilst their values were different to hers, that was okay. This shift Hannah chose to make had positive consequences almost immediately and caused their relationship to grow stronger and more supportive of one another, which was the quality of family connectedness that Hannah had been longing to experience for many years.

*Pursuing your soul's desire triggers
a process of internal alchemy that
is sensed before it's observed
and understood.*

SOUL SUMMARY

- Your soul speaks to you in subtle whispers; it's called intuition.
- Allowing your soul to guide your decisions keeps you on track towards the life experiences that would be most beneficial for your overall development.
- Your soul can choose to pursue experiences in life that enable you to learn, grow and evolve.
- Your soul's mission in having a human life is to gain wisdom through its experiences.
- The greater your soul's wisdom the more understanding and appreciation you have for how intricately connected you are to all life.
- Your soul evolves through your intentions and the choices you make.
- The soul's greatest desires are love and wisdom.

3 ways to reveal your soul's desire

- Develop your intuition. Pay attention to its subtle persistent whispers and signs guiding you to explore a subject, person, place, event or thing more thoroughly.
- Dive into subjects you're consistently drawn to (or interested in), and pay attention if these energise and inspire you.
- Notice what you're avoiding or what causes you frustration, anger or sadness. Emotional hooks are also clues. Consider what the contrasting experience might feel and look like and take steps in that direction.

You attract what's best when you're 100 per cent yourself.

Chapter Seven

KEY 2: AUTHENTICITY

KEY 2: AUTHENTICITY

Authenticity means honouring your feelings, expressing your truth and doing what's right for you. Standing with your soul's unique form of self-expression is your power-place.

When you're inauthentic you can feel disconnected, uninspired and fatigued. Finding your authentic self can be challenging, especially if you allow others to decide what's right for you. The vibrational frequencies of authenticity feel good in your mind *and* body.

Is your social media persona idealised on Facebook, Instagram, Twitter or dating profiles? Everyone's life can look glamorous and exciting for five minutes a day, but it's important to remember that it's not reality; it's a snapshot of someone's life. What you post may seem harmless to you on a conscious level, but could be having an unsupportive effect on you unconsciously in maintaining your authenticity.

Every time you choose authenticity you're developing self-trust. When your self-trust is high, you don't feel the need to justify decisions. It also draws like-minded authentic people to you and makes it easier for you to maintain healthy boundaries in relationships by helping you to recognise when you are losing yourself, trying to please other people. Authentic power comes from feeling that what you're doing is right for you – it's a strong gut feeling that you're meeting *your* needs.

Living authentically is like standing directly under your soul's spotlight; fully illuminated and energised by it. Imagine stepping out of that spotlight, to the right or left. You can still be seen, but you're partly shadowed.

Next time you decide to please someone over yourself, notice how quickly your body expresses resistance to your decision. Moving away from your authenticity has an instant depleting effect on your energy and can even result in building resentment towards that person, especially if you've had to dial yourself down to be accepted.

Being your authentic self isn't an excuse for being insensitive to others. It's worth remembering that just because people you care about disagree with you doesn't mean they don't respect, care and love you.

Returning to the authentic self

To find our way back to our authentic self, we need to develop our level of self-awareness to recognise who we are choosing to be from moment to moment and how that is affecting the quality of life we are experiencing. With self-awareness we can more easily catch ourselves when what we are thinking, saying or doing is moving us away from who we know ourselves to be. The energetic contrast of being in our authenticity or out of it is easily felt when we are self-aware. The out-of-authenticity state can often feel like a loss of personal power and energy. In contrast when we are our authentic selves we feel empowered and energised. By remaining vigilant of this contrasting experience we can act quickly when we feel we are moving away from who we truly are.

There might be other societal pressures on you to be something *that isn't authentically what feels right for you.* Perhaps your life turned out in a way you didn't plan. You may have convinced yourself to be:

- In a family business
- The breadwinner
- A stay-at-home parent
- Subservient to your partner by sacrificing your own needs
- A social drinker just so your friends feel comfortable when they drink
- In the closet about your same-sex attraction
- Passive when people you socialise with share judgemental opinions

Can you recall meeting a person who you instantly felt was genuine and transparent with you? You may not have realised it, but it's highly likely that your intuition was giving you that energetic feedback about them. The frequencies that your body receives and broadcasts from your thoughts and feelings is also being broadcast and received by everyone else as well (whether they're aware of it or not). The saying, *trust your first impressions* has lots of merit. Often before our analytical mind gets in the way, we receive an intuitive impulse about someone. When that person's energy field (comprised of their beliefs, thoughts, language and actions) also resonates with yours, you might find you immediately relax in their company.

Conversely, when you pick up that a person's ideas or desires are diametrically opposed to yours, you might start to feel uncomfortable around them; you may even find them disingenuous. As you *sense* them they can sense you. Your body plays out the feedback from your intuition, regardless of what face you show the world. Think about that next time you attend an interview, ask someone out on a date, have a disagreement or are working to close a deal.

Being yourself is always the most powerful energetic position you can occupy. If being authentic and true means you don't get the job, the gal, the guy, the house, the deal or the cash from your friends or family, then let it go. It wasn't meant to be. Another opportunity will present itself, or perhaps it's a sign that you need to review your plans. When you move out of your authenticity to get what you *think* you want, or tell someone what they want to hear, you're inviting disharmony into your life.

AUTHENTICITY IS ESSENTIAL

Every relationship you have is built on the quality of the relationship you have with yourself. **That's worth re-reading.**

When you're patient, compassionate, nurturing, kind and connected to yourself, you'll behave that way towards people in your life. If your soul's desire involves attracting a partner, improving relationships with family or friends or resolving issues with your existing partner, you'll gain strides by improving the relationship with yourself first. Love is connection. It's practice, not theory.

If you tell yourself you need someone in your life to make it better you are focusing on *lack*, which doesn't feel good. Energetically speaking, unsupportive feelings are low-awareness states that broadcast unsupportive vibrational frequencies into your environment and attract more of what you're trying to get away from. For instance, being alone doesn't mean being lonely. If you develop self-love and self-acceptance, you'll become comfortable in your own company and you'll find periods of solitude enjoyable and restorative.

Solitude is *not* loneliness. One is by choice, the other is not. When you tell yourself you're lonely, but in reality you're not as you have people that love and care for you within reach, you'll go looking for distractions. You may find yourself frequently drawn to places that other lonely people frequently go to, like casinos, bars or to online dating sites to secure a permanent partner or do anything that puts you amongst people to fill that perceived void. When you believe you're lonely, nothing you can do for yourself, or what anyone can do for you, will be enough to satisfy you. It's like a permanent itch that needs scratching.

When you *believe* you're lonely you're likely to load expectations onto your relationships, which can result in tension. *Expectations* are connected to concerns around lack or loss. Holding those kinds of beliefs and thoughts has a lowering effect on the vibrational frequencies you're broadcasting; it decreases your energy levels instantly and can make you feel down. Conversely, when you focus on releasing expectations and look for the goodness in your relationships – no matter how small and you choose not to go back to any unsupportive patterns of behaviour – you are choosing to move to a elevated level of awareness. This choice means you'll broadcast a higher vibrational frequency, and so long as you maintain alignment to the desire to have a great relationship with any person, it now has the opportunity to improve.

Everyday Miracle Makers know their daily work is about learning when and how to shift the vibrational frequency of their beliefs, thoughts, actions and language to bring them into alignment with what they desire. If you want to be in a relationship, but that special person just isn't showing up, it's a sign that you're out of harmony with what you desire. You don't need to go searching for the right person; just focus your attention on creating vibrational alignment and they'll appear. You can do that by ensuring what you believe, think, do and say about wanting to be in a relationship are in agreement. If you discover any opposition in any of these aspects of yourself, work to turn them around to achieve alignment. When you do this, you will be astounded at how fast the right person can 'coincidentally' show up.

WHY BOUNDARIES ARE IMPORTANT

Being in touch with your authenticity makes it easier to maintain boundaries, especially with the people you care about the most.

If you can't be who you really are around people you love (or have to tippy-toe your truth around them in case it upsets them), your intuition has probably been whispering to you that the relationship needs balance. Intuition is subtle, but its silent nudges can keep demanding your attention.

I've heard many clients say that they often suppress their thoughts and feelings to keep the peace in their family. Keep in mind if you do this regularly you're moving away from your authenticity. Being authentic means at some point you'll experience rejection because you aren't changing who you are to suit how somebody else wants you to be. People who are emotionally mature or have healthy self-esteem tend to be clear communicators; these people can agree to disagree with you without it affecting your relationship with them.

Your decision to do what feels right for you might shatter some illusions for other people and what they expect of you, but that's theirs to resolve.

There are lots of clues to listen out for when you are outside your authenticity. All of the following behaviours set up a cycle that's difficult to free yourself from:

- Attempting to keep the peace
- Faking what you think and how you feel
- Looking for regular validation from others
- People-pleasing
- Giving compliments to be liked
- Picking up the bill every time you go out with people to be perceived as financially successful

The longer you continue to deny your true self, the deeper it affects your self-esteem. People with healthy self-esteem don't fear rejection around pleasing others. If you've ever felt that your parents/partner/family don't understand or get you, consider that it might be you're not being your authentic self around them, and they can feel a discord with you.

If you feel you need to reclaim your authenticity, do it. Start by taking one small step today to bring yourself back into alignment with who you really are; *all* your relationships will benefit from it, one way or another.

Locating your authentic self takes practice and courage. Physically you can disguise your true self with clothing or make-up, or personality traits that aren't really you.

When we choose to let go of what people think of us, and drop any facades we've created about ourselves and end the pursuit of doing what we think we should be doing (or having), then we move closer to regaining our authenticity.

If you feel like you were on the path to your soul's desire, but after experiencing a couple of life's knocks, you've fallen into a hole you can't climb out of, try this exercise.

Everyday Miracle Maker Exercise: Reclaiming your authentic self

Visualise a stage with a bright white spotlight shining down. Imagine yourself standing directly beneath it. This scene represents the brilliance of you living your life authentically, expressing and radiating your soul's light. Now mentally project an image of yourself into the shadow area just outside of the spotlight. This is just a mental projection. Our minds can create and activate a projected self into any environment at our command. It can happen when we feel insecure and perceive that being someone else is better than being ourselves; we think it'll make us more acceptable because the real us isn't good enough. For most people this projected-self gets switched on in certain situations or around certain people. But for others, the projected-self stays switched on most of the time.

Over time we can start to loose touch with who we really are and what is right and true for us. This happens because we lose contact with the energetic feedback of what the *real* us thinks, feels and knows. The projected-self also depletes the physical body and mind of energy because a projection has no capacity to store or generate energy of its own.

So, how do you find your way back to your real self where the light of your soul shines the brightest? Trust that you know what's best for you. No matter how much you love, care or respect a person giving you advice, start by making decisions for yourself that feel right for you. Choose to release concern around what others may think of you. When you do this consistently and deliberately your mind and body will find its way back beneath the spotlight where you'll feel re-energised by your soul's power.

Being outside of your comfort zone

Sometimes making a certain decision doesn't feel right for us because we can perceive that to pursue it we would be acting outside of our authenticity, but it isn't. For instance, when learning new skills we can feel vulnerable because we're being challenged by something unfamiliar and this can create mental and physical discomfort. On these occasions check in with yourself because maybe what's been asked of you is just outside your comfort zone. For example, if you're offered the opportunity to upskill at work and that includes public speaking (one of people's biggest fears) understand that the discomfort you feel could be your fear of speaking in front of a group (rather than feeling the job is not right for you). To grow we need to keep expanding our comfort zones. We're all works in progress. Who you knew yourself to be 10 years ago is different to the person who you are today. Your likes and dislikes change and your authenticity morphs with those changes.

*Identify the person you need to be
in your inner and outer world
to experience mental peace and
emotional comfort; you'll find
authenticity there.*

EVERYDAY MIRACLE MAKER EXAMPLE – AUTHENTICITY

Name: Julie

Age: 39

Julie had low self-esteem.

She had lost her ability to make decisions on her own, even simple ones like which laundry detergent to buy. When her relationship ended, it shattered the remnants of her self-esteem; after years of living with an unsupportive partner she was at rock bottom.

Julie said that her self-esteem was at its lowest when she communicated with her ex. Even though she'd enjoyed her job when she first started out, she'd stayed with the company because her ex-partner wanted her to. The money was good and she also convinced herself that she wasn't confident enough to handle interviews for senior roles anywhere else, let alone pursue her soul's desire. Her ex-partner's success in business made her feel that they knew what was best for her. It wasn't.

I helped Julie to understand that our self-esteem is directly connected to our authenticity. When we ignore the feelings of what's right for us and make decisions surrounding our life to please others, we can loose touch with ourselves. When we do what's right for us we feel aligned, cohesive, valued and powerful. Though she knew deep down that her ex-partner's control over her life wasn't right and she'd allowed it, she didn't know how to begin changing it.

Introducing the concepts of authenticity and energy increases and decreases to Julie made a huge difference to her life. When someone close to her (or in a perceived position of influence) placed demands on her, whether it was as seemingly small as attending a social event, she now paused and thought about it, instead of instantly saying yes and regretting the decision later. She began to understand that when she honoured how she felt, she valued herself more and knew it was building her self-esteem.

Every time Julie stepped away from her authenticity to be someone that other people wanted her to be, she felt energetically depleted because she was choosing, consciously or not, lower frequency beliefs and thoughts. She was sending a signal to her unconscious mind that what she wanted wasn't as important as meeting the needs of other people and this was affecting her self-esteem. It was an a-ha moment for her; until then she didn't understand that they were connected.

Our unconscious mind *believes* us. If we're constantly telling it that other people's needs are more important than ours, it'll diminish our self-esteem. We worked on ways she could say no kindly to those around her, or thank them, without feeling pressure or beholden to take their advice.

Julie's self-esteem increased, she was re-energised about her life and chose to leave her job. She became assertive about expressing herself around her ex and started her own business focused on a soul's desire.

When you're inauthentic it's energy depleting, when you're authentic it's energising.

AUTHENTICITY SUMMARY

- Authenticity is being true to yourself and who you know yourself to be.
- Express your likes, dislikes, beliefs, preferences and opinions and show the world the real you.
- Being authentic is your power-place because it is your soul's unique form of self-expression.
- Honouring your authenticity makes it easier to maintain boundaries, especially with people you care about the most.
- Trust that you're the best person to know what's right for you.
- When you move away from your authenticity you'll experience a decrease in energy.
- Authenticity is unbiased self-awareness.

3 ways to reclaim your authenticity

- Develop your self-awareness in order to recognise when you are being different to who you truly know yourself to be.
- Identify and communicate boundaries in your relationships. It might mean letting your partner know that even though they love and care for you, *you* know what's best for you.
- Stop worrying about what people think of you and instead improve your relationship with yourself. Love and accept yourself now for who you are.

When you can't see it, sense it.

Chapter Eight

KEY 3: INTUITION

KEY 3: INTUITION

Intuition is the voice of your soul. It's available 24/7 unprompted and on command when you focus your attention on how you *feel* about something.

Your heart and gut are sensitive gauges of intuitive guidance and will always offer you vibrational feedback. The type of sensations the vibrational feedback evokes, whether positive or negative, supportive or not, is information you can use to move towards, or away from any decision.

Intuition is higher than instinct. Instinct *protects* you; intuition *guides* you. Whether you call intuition your inner voice, a gut feeling or a hunch, the spectrum of intelligent information you can access by developing your intuition can astound you.

You're a walking, talking, sending and receiving tower of vibrational frequencies. When you deliberately and regularly practise tuning in to your body's intuitive communication system, you'll develop your skills to increasingly higher levels of competency. As you do, you gain knowledge beyond memories that are stored in your unconscious mind. My three decades of research, personal knowledge and experience has taught me that the level of intelligence we can access through our intuition is limitless.

When emotions run high, you're often driven by instinct, not intuition. Intuition provides a greater perspective than the lower reaches of your analytical mind (which leans towards activity and anxiety, rather than calm and centredness). Intuitive impulses are best described by your intellect than explained by it, the reason being intuition is superior to intellect. However you need the analytical mind in order to work with intuition.

Your intuition sources information from many places including; memories stored in your unconscious mind, your imagination, through your soul and via other influences. Depending on the level of your intuitive development, your intuition can tune into information about people, places, events and things and isn't constrained by time, space or any retained information.

Learning how to better interpret your intuition takes practice, but it's a skill anyone can learn. If your intuition guides you about something, stay true to what you feel. Pressing the 'Intuition Override' button is not a good idea (but I'm sensing you already know that).

Your body's intuitive communication system includes your ability to sense, feel, know, see, smell and hear information about any subject you focus your attention on. Some of the ways you can receive answers are as a thought, a feeling or an image. Have you ever felt quietly confident a situation was going to turn out well and it did, yet you had no objective evidence to support that feeling? That was your intuition speaking to you.

Intuition has its naysayers; sceptics who dismiss 'gut feelings' as sentimental overreactions to situations. But intuition isn't just a 21st century buzzword. Oracles and medicine people throughout history have espoused the virtues of higher states of mind – from the Babylonians to the Buddhists, the Hindus to the Hebrews. Globally there's been an understanding in many cultures that there's something sensible about having a sixth sense.

In 350 B.C. philosopher and scientist Aristotle formally recognised the power of perception and sensation. He described wisdom as being a combination of intuitive reason and scientific knowledge, early proof that there was something deeper to hunches. Early 20th century philosophers and psychiatrists like Carl Jung wrote extensively about intuitiveness. He stated that humans view the world through four ways: feeling, sensation, thinking and intuition.

You can gain insight on how to transform any challenge just by engaging your intuition. By sending and receiving vibrational frequencies your intuition is able to provide you with feedback about a person, place, event or thing. Your intuitive impulses will either feel supportive, *neutral* or unsupportive. Using intuition means you're tuning into a higher level of intelligence than normal conscious awareness.

Intuition is at its best and most accurate when you're calm and relaxed.

MAKE BETTER DECISIONS

Intuition is a scientifically recognised psychological phenomenon.

Some of the greatest decisions in history have come from those who valued their intuition; Steve Jobs, Albert Einstein and Pablo Picasso have credited their intuition with some of their best career choices. Developing your intuition together with your imagination and creativity is priceless.

Despite intuitive cheerleaders like that, many new clients I work with can still be apprehensive to use it; many people don't trust their intuition and often say it isn't reliable for them. Intuition is a skill and like all skills it can be upgraded and improved upon.

Have you ever liked or disliked a person the moment you met them and didn't know why? It could be because of the intuitive feedback you were unconsciously receiving. Or it could have been that the person's looks or behaviour was familiar to you in some way that you weren't conscious of and misinterpreted it as intuitive feedback. Regardless of whether the feeling is positive or negative we can develop an immediate bias, without realising it.

Next time you have to make a decision, be discerning around whether you are being influenced by an existing bias about people, places, events or things or whether it's your intuition speaking to you. Given that most people favour mental reasoning over intuition in decision making to arrive at a holistic decision it is important to realise we need to use both.

We're all born with an inner sense, just like we were born to float, but learning to swim takes practice. So does developing your intuition. If your intuition offered you help in the past, whether you've listened to it or not, it's a sign that you should consider developing your intuitive ability.

Everyday Miracle Makers use their intuition regularly to solve challenges and identify opportunities for themselves, their families, communities and organisations.

*Your intuition knows what you
need, even when you think you
know what you want.*

EVERYDAY MIRACLE MAKER EXAMPLE - INTUITION

Name: Marcus

Age: 56

Marcus' landscaping business was failing.

It was his soul's desire, but he constantly attracted late-paying customers, which was affecting his ability to make ends meet.

He suffered from insomnia and his creditors were constantly on his back. Employing debt collectors only relieved the stress momentarily; it wasn't long before another debt was in play. Marcus couldn't understand why he was attracting what he called bad luck, and employing lawyers to enforce payment clauses in the contracts he signed with developers was an expense he couldn't afford.

I asked Marcus if he trusted his gut feelings about people and situations and despite him saying yes, he said he also rarely acted on them. In fact, some late-paying clients all gave him feelings of discomfort before signing contracts, but he took them on board because the profit was good which caused him to move out of alignment. The stress and disruption it had caused to his business and relationship was now not worth it.

I explained to Marcus that we often override our intuition when we convince ourselves that what we hope to gain is more valuable than listening to this higher guidance. The only way Marcus could turn this around was to upgrade his relationship with his intuition and start living by more supportive behaviours.

Four months after my sessions with Marcus ended he called me to say that he'd accepted two new contracts and rejected another two, because his gut was telling him something wasn't right. He requested additional security around payment, but the clauses were rebuffed. Turns out the two contracts he rejected based on his intuitive alerts would have sunk him. Marcus was surprised how much had changed for him since tuning in to and valuing his intuitive guidance in his decision-making process. His confidence, business and relationship were back in alignment and growing.

If you don't trust your intuition enough to follow it, it's not your intuition you're listening to.

INTUITION SUMMARY

- Intuition is your soul's guidance. It's available 24/7 unprompted and on command.

- It's higher than instinct. Instinct protects you; intuition guides you.

- Your heart and gut are sensitive gauges for intuitive guidance.

- Intuition is an invaluable tool for fast and holistic decision-making.

- When you develop and practise tuning in to your intuition you can access valuable insight on any situation in your life.

- Keep your mind open; answers to intuitive questions can appear in many ways.

- The intellect can be used to describe intuition, but not explain it, because intuition is superior to intellect.

3 ways to develop your intuition

- Broaden your scope of attention. Recognise that your intuition might be communicating to you in more ways than you are currently open to. For instance; through conversations, a piece of music, a character in a television show, a bumper sticker or something as seemingly random as a piece of graffiti you're drawn to read.

- Meditate for 15+ minutes a day to invite the connection to your soul's guidance. Meditation helps you withdraw from the visible world and move into the invisible world. The silence creates a retreat for your mind, and replenishes and educates it to become sensitive to communication from the soul's realm where answers can drop in.

- Ask a question before falling asleep and take notes if your answer is played out in your dreams. Keep a record of questions you put to your intuition in your journal. Keep questions to your intuition uncomplicated. For instance, *"What learning do I need to focus on from this experience to move forward with ease?"* Or you may choose to turn the question into a statement. Use whichever approach gets you the best results.

Look forward to what you want to be, do or have without overlooking the value of the present moment.

Chapter Nine

KEY 4: GRATITUDE

KEY 4: GRATITUDE

Giving gratitude is recognition that goodness has and is showing up in your life, and you have many things to be thankful for now. Gratitude is an amplifying frequency that is broadcast from our heart centre and allows us to penetrate a larger reality with our mind than the limited material world. Appreciation enhances your ability to attract abundance in what you value, whether it has manifested in your life or has yet to.

When you make it a regular practice to express gratitude for what you have and what you've accomplished, you are choosing a higher state of awareness and this attracts more everyday miracles to show up in your life to be grateful for. There are always things in your life you can offer gratitude for, but you need to be willing to recognise them. I also recommend giving gratitude for things that don't go your way and with the benefit of hindsight, you're glad that they didn't.

The gratitude you express might relate to:

- Thinking more supportive thoughts and how much happier you feel.
- Arguing less with your partner and wanting to be together more often.
- Demonstrating discipline around meditating more often and feeling centred and peaceful by it.
- Finding an opportunity to laugh everyday.

- Being recognised at work for a project and feeling delighted with your contribution.

- Sleeping through the night and waking refreshed.

- Having days where your body feels less pained and more mobile allowing you to enjoy the activities you love.

- Your ability to be childlike and maintain your wonderment and curiosity with the world around you.

- The opportunity to give back to your parents or grandparents for supporting you.

- Overcoming nervousness to attend a networking event on your own and making valuable contacts.

- Your house not selling when first put on the market and when you relisted it later the market was at an all-time high.

- Your ex refusing your plea to get back together and six months later you meet your soul mate.

Think of the most grateful and appreciative person you know – can you recall how good you feel in their company? You feel this way because the energetic exchange you have with them is energising and expanding to your energy field. Conversely, now think about someone else who is rarely grateful or appreciative for anything in his or her life. Can you feel the vibrational contrast in your body just by visiting each of these people's overall vibrational frequency with your mind? You don't need a device to measure the intensity of what feels good and what doesn't; your intelligent energy body will give you the feedback in seconds.

Everyday Miracle Makers practise gratitude and appreciation daily because they know it has the effect of energetically enhancing every dimension of their life; it's like putting drops of pink dye into a tank of clear water. The tank water represents the energy of your body and mind, and every 'I'm grateful for...' is like adding a drop of pink dye to the water. Eventually, the dye will occupy every corner of the tank and turn the water pink. You don't have to fill the entire tank with pink drops, you just have to release enough drops of dye into the water for the flow-on effect to occur. That's what gratitude does; it seeps into and enhances all dimensions of your life.

When you say 'thank you', make it specific. Also be thankful for beliefs, thoughts and feelings that you've noticed have undergone a frequency shift and are now supportive. Feel the appreciation. Allow it to expand throughout every part of your body until you're overflowing with gratitude.

SUCCESSFULLY BANISH NEGATIVITY

In all our interactions choice-points exist. These are the moments between what *happens,* what we make it *mean* and how we choose to *respond* to it.

You're always deciding whether something is positive or negative, good or bad, helpful or disruptive. What *you* decide is a result of your existing beliefs about that person, place, event or thing. If you're experiencing a situation that routinely makes you feel lousy, ask yourself how you're contributing to making it unsupportive. Challenge how you're thinking about it and find something to be grateful for to shift your frequency up from the basement to the penthouse. The view is always nicer from up high…

Everything you say to yourself matters. When you're thinking and speaking kindly and supportively of yourself, you're practising self-care and that higher frequency draws quality experiences, opportunities and like-minded people to you. If you ever become aware that you're beating yourself up or having a pity party for one, say out loud, 'STOP'. This helps you recognise when you're in a loop of negativity and hits the brakes to disrupt your unsupportive thinking. This creates a choice-point where you can select an alternative thought that is healthier and more helpful for your wellbeing.

HOW TO STAY PRESENT

Self-awareness is your ability to know what's going on in your mind, body and the environment around you.

You become the most self-aware when you bring your focus to the present moment. "Presence" increases mental peace, but like any new skill it'll take practice and commitment to develop. When you condition your mind to keep returning to the present moment in time it will follow your orders with less effort.

One of the easiest ways to be fully present is by being totally engaged in what you're doing. If you're cooking, keep your thoughts on what you're making; even read the recipe out loud. Put loving thoughts into the food and think about who you're cooking it for. If you're going for a walk stay engaged in the moment by looking at the trees, the sky and the environment around you and be grateful for the beauty of nature. Notice the details of the trees, plants or buildings, and be aware of the feeling of the soles of your feet walking on the ground that will keep you in the present moment.

More effective ways to become self-aware and bring your thoughts back to your body are to:

- Take off your shoes and let the soles of your feet touch grass, the earth or beach sand.
- Go swimming.
- Interact with your pets.
- Moisturise your hands and/or body and do it lovingly.
- Inhale through your nose counting to 4, hold for a second then exhale counting to 6 (repeat 4x).

Everyday Miracle Maker Exercise: Thinking, Feeling and Energy

Picture a pyramid. Its apex (highest point) represents now – the present. It's the place where your thoughts are calm, your body feels relaxed and your energy is balanced.

Now, mentally travel down the left side of the pyramid, this represents recollections – the past. Any recollection you have that makes you feel down is unsupportive. The longer you dwell on that type of thought no matter if it occurred yesterday or years ago, the worse you can feel. This relationship also decreases the amount of energy (vitality) you experience in your body.

This time mentally travel down the right side of the pyramid, this represents expectations – the future. Any expectation you have that makes you feel anxious is also unsupportive. Whether it's associated with an event to occur in hours, days or years from now, you'll become anxious and nervous the longer you dwell on it. For example, a phone call catch up with a friend or client has just been changed by them to a meeting over coffee instead. As long as you choose to interpret this event change as neutral or positive, you will maintain your existing thinking feeling relationship and will continue feeling good and shouldn't experience a drop in your energy level. However, if you begin generating expectations that the event change from a phone call to in person, is because they have bad news and you dwelled on that unsupportive expectation, it can make you anxious. This thinking feeling relationship also has the effect of decreasing the amount of energy you experience in your body.

Not all recollections and expectations you have decrease your energy levels. You'll notice when you recollect a situation from your past you feel happy about, it can have the opposite effect. Also, when you visualise how you'll feel accomplishing your Soul's Desire in the future this expectation can make you feel pumped, full of energy and excited.

This exercise is designed to help you recognise there's a relationship between what you're thinking and how you're feeling and the energy level you experience. When you become increasingly aware of this connection you can act quickly to upgrade and/or neutralise your thoughts to improve how you feel which can increase your energy level immediately.

→ *Check out the Thinking, Feeling and Energy Pyramid on page 190.*

Gratitude comes from the heart.
It's valuable shown and spoken.

EVERYDAY MIRACLE MAKER EXAMPLE – GRATITUDE

Name: David:

Age: 45

David was in significant physical pain. He had pain in his right shoulder and in his thoracic area (directly behind the heart centre). He had x-rays, saw medical professionals, but there wasn't enough relief for David that he could return to work. He told me he felt *frozen* and was on high levels of pain medication.

David was a single parent supporting his children. He had help from his parents with the kids and household, but he couldn't take much more time off work without compromising his position with his father who heavily depended on him in his business.

I suggested we work on trying to shift the pain by shifting (raising) the frequency of those areas of his body, specifically where the pain and lack of movement was most severe.

Before I continued, I asked David to rate the pain so we could determine if there was a shift. On a scale of 1 out of 10 the pain in the centre of his spine directly behind his heart centre was 8 out of 10. The pain and discomfort in his right shoulder was 7 out of 10.

Four months earlier David had become 'super stressed' – he wanted to leave his father's plumbing business to pursue his passion of renovating and selling properties, but every time he'd discussed leaving, his father shut him down.

David felt stuck. He felt that because he was his father's right arm in the business he was guilt-tripped into staying.

It's no surprise that David was experiencing pain in his right shoulder. I explained that our bodies can express what our minds can no longer repress. Our persistent thoughts have the power to produce a positive or negative effect in our bodies.

David and I worked on upgrading his existing beliefs. I asked him if he would be willing to release and upgrade his beliefs about his father as that could have a positive effect on his energy field and his physical body. He agreed.

I showed David how he could express gratitude instead of bitterness towards him by referencing positive facts about their relationship that were supportive and suggested focusing on that instead.

I also asked David to take his awareness to his right shoulder and thank his father for allowing him to be his right-hand man. I encouraged him to acknowledge the financial support and opportunities he received while working for him.

By the end of the first session, both areas of pain had decreased by three to four points and were now sitting at 4-5 out of 10. He was astounded by the knock-on effect of expressing gratitude to his father.

Within three days, David reported that the pain had subsided to a 2. He was back at work and feeling stronger than he'd done in a long time. He thanked his father and talked with him about moving on and this time stood firm in his decision to leave. Unexpectedly for David, his father wished him well, and his phased exit from the business was implemented.

The simplest meditations are often the most powerful.

I am grateful for _____ .
(Fill in the blank).

GRATITUDE SUMMARY

- To experience gratitude as a feeling, hold it as an intention and focus your attention at your heart centre.

- Practising gratitude keeps you aligned to the vibrational frequencies of abundance.

- When you say 'thank you' make it specific. Feel the appreciation and allow it to amplify from your heart throughout your entire body.

- If you're experiencing an event that makes you feel lousy, make a U-turn and mentally go in the opposite direction and find something to be grateful for; you'll quickly experience a frequency shift and a more supportive emotional state.

- Practising gratitude often cues your unconscious mind to know this experience is important to you and it will work to help you draw more experiences into your life to be grateful for.

- Gratitude is an amplifying vibrational frequency.

3 ways to practise gratitude

- Connect with a thought or speak aloud how grateful you are for parts of your daily routine that you love. For instance, a well-made cup of tea, delicious meal, a refreshing swim, an energising workout or time spent with those you love and care about.

- Be grateful for what *hasn't* shown up in your physical world yet. Speak about it in the *present tense*. Convince your unconscious mind it already exists energetically and it's only a matter of time before you experience it physically.

- Before drifting off to sleep each night, imagine mentally writing three gratitude notes to people who enhanced your experience of the day by telling them *specifically* why you're so grateful to them. You can also send a gratitude note to your pet, and a specific location in nature or anywhere in the cosmos for that matter. I also recommend extending gratitude to the highest power you recognise. This reinforces to your unconscious mind that you're aware you are always being supported. Giving gratitude to a higher power also helps keep our ego in check.

When what you believe, think,
do and say are in agreement,
you're in alignment.

Chapter Ten

KEY 5: ALIGNMENT

KEY 5: ALIGNMENT

Alignment is being in agreement. When your beliefs, thoughts, actions and language reinforce each other – you're aligned. This produces a feeling of certainty that you're on the right path and that all your energy is travelling in the same direction.

When they do you're on the fast track to accomplishment.

Everyday Miracle-Making is about being (and staying) aligned. When you're aligned you expand the feeling of certainty that you're on the right path and trust in the direction you're heading.

To achieve alignment you need to take ownership for all areas of your life, including the areas you find unattractive or difficult. People who experience success in many areas of their life often do so because they choose to participate in every dimension of their life whether they want to or not, because they know the payoff is worth it. If you don't have what you want yet, identify what aspect of yourself (beliefs, thoughts, actions or language) is contradictory to accomplishing your soul's desire. By renewing your commitment and taking new action to bring all aspects of yourself into agreement this will result in the frequency shift you need to achieve alignment to your soul's desire.

What can get in the way of achieving alignment:

- Attending job interviews, yet thinking it's unlikely you'll secure a job soon.

- Thinking you want to improve the relationship with your partner, yet you deliberately withdraw from them mentally, emotionally and physically.

- Believing you're ready to meet your soul mate, yet you repeat phrases like 'there is no one out there for me'.

- Saying you want more in your life to be grateful for, yet not giving gratitude for what you already have.

- Thoroughly researching a business idea, yet not believing you know enough to get started.

- Knowing the relationship you're in isn't right, but staying in it because you don't want to be alone.

- Communicating that you want to build a profitable business, yet showing little discipline in managing expenses.

- Wanting your partner to be more financially responsible, yet you continue to make all the financial decisions.

Everyday Miracle Makers know that achieving and maintaining alignment is pivotal in closing the gap between where they are and arriving at their soul's desire. When you make a conscious daily commitment to practise alignment, what you need will appear from the invisible world into the visible to surprise and delight you.

I'm often asked, is it enough to focus exclusively on the key of alignment? My answer is always no. History has many examples of individuals who were totally aligned to negative outcomes that caused harm. For this reason practising the other 6 keys along with alignment is important and ensures you'll cultivate the optimal vibrational atmosphere to attract positive and loving experiences into your life and the lives of others.

If being wealthy is your soul's desire and you haven't accomplished it yet, perhaps you're avoiding some of the dimensions to building wealth. Everday Miracle Makers build wealth by adopting a perspective that their wealth can *help* them do more to help others. When your money works for you, you'll have more freedom to choose the work you want to do.

The better-known dimensions around building holistic wealth are having a consistent source of income, keeping expenses lower than earnings, saving and investing. Charitable giving also helps build wealth. When we give more we become wealthier and with increased wealth we give more. However, unless your beliefs, thoughts, actions and language support this soul's desire, you're likely to struggle. Let me explain. Say you want to be wealthy, but you still hold beliefs that you don't need to give up anything that gives you pleasure like, overseas holidays, buying designer clothes and shoes anytime you feel like it, or going to expensive restaurants – nothing will change. As a result you have little money to save, none to invest and you may find yourself in debt. *If you spend most of your money you'll be qualified at spending money not building wealth.* Believing you want to be wealthy and speaking about it is not enough, to achieve alignment your thoughts and actions must be congruent with your beliefs and language around building wealth.

Remember, energy does not discriminate; it draws likeness together and separates what isn't. Getting closer to building wealth is achievable when you choose to neutralise any opposition you are creating around it. Beliefs are deeper than thoughts; they sit in our unconscious mind and drive our behaviour.

It takes self-responsibility and discipline to save money and it can feel like hard work if you're secretly wishing you didn't have to do it. Make it easier for yourself and decide it isn't going to be difficult. Instead it's going to be an adventure. Turn it into a game and challenge yourself to see how well you can do.

Have you set numerous goals you haven't accomplished? If you have, it's time to forgive yourself and take a fresh approach towards them.

The Everyday Miracle Maker is not a wishful thinker; she or he takes deliberate action to move themselves towards their soul's desire. Everyday Miracle Makers see themselves as students of life and are always willing to learn and do what needs to be done to progress.

THE GOOD LUCK SLIPSTREAM

Have you ever experienced a stream of good luck? It could be something like, finding car parking spaces all day, or looking for work and bumping into a former colleague and they offer you a job, or leaving an expensive umbrella on a busy commuter train on the way to work and finding it on the trip home later that evening. That's you unconsciously generating what I call, the Slipstream Effect.

The Slipstream Effect brings people, places, events and things into your life rapidly when you're in an optimal frequency state. It's a flurry of everyday miracles.

If you've ever watched a flock of migrating birds in a V formation, or seen a pack of cyclists on the road riding 30cm apart they're benefiting from the leader's slipstream. Air flows behind the frontrunners so the birds (or cyclists) at the back take advantage of the slipstream; they save on the energy they need to expend. When you choose to learn and live the 7 self-transformation keys to unlock your miracle-making mindset, you can trigger the energetic equivalent of the slipstream. During this period of time you can experience everyday miracles in such rapid succession that it can be jaw dropping. It could be that your phone rings and the crazy offer you put on a car is accepted, you're invited on a date by someone you really like, there's a sudden shift in your health for the better and your energy levels have returned, or while walking down the street a $100 bill tumbles towards you with no one in sight.

Remind yourself that your soul's desire has an invisible component that needs to be fulfilled energetically. Commit to increasing the frequency of your beliefs, thoughts, actions and language when you identify that you are feeling some resistance or disharmony. This will keep you moving in the right direction towards your soul's desire.

ALIGNMENT AND TEAMS

Whilst *Everyday Miracle Maker* has been written as a guide to self-transformation for individuals, the 7 self-transformation keys can be applied to teams in any business and organisation. I have been drawing on the keys in my work with Managing Directors, CEOs and senior executives across many industries who work with their teams in transformation projects. When leaders invite the level of awareness suggested in *Everyday Miracle Maker* into their organisations to transform culture, products and services to better serve people and planet, we all win.

Having worked in small, medium and large companies, I observed many high performing teams. That reminded me of specific coaching sessions when clients shared they felt internal resistance to business goals. Feeling resistance is a sign you're out of alignment to the goal. Sometimes you can be unconsciously out of alignment, meaning you don't realise that what you're believing, thinking or doing is getting in the way of you achieving the desired results. Other times it's in the form of conscious resistance. For example, you disagree with the goal or the approach you are being asked to take and you're aware it's affecting your performance in achieving it. Whether the resistance is conscious or unconscious many clients have shared they experience an increase in stress, and a decrease in work satisfaction, the longer they allow their out of alignment state to continue. Conversely, when alignment is achieved the opposite occurs, they feel happier at work immediately which has an impact on their productivity and performance.

If you've ever found yourself in a situation like this or you're a leader who is interested in supporting your team to achieve optimal outcomes for the business, I suggest you keep alignment top of mind.

THE SELF-TALK BOARDWALK

Your self-talk could be counter-productive to what you want to accomplish. You may want it, but not *believe* you can have it or accomplish it.

If your unconscious beliefs are doubtful you'll experience energy blocks. These blocks interfere with the flow of subtle energy throughout your body and often get in the way of you moving forward in a helpful way. Start by choosing better, more supportive and gentler feelings, beliefs and thoughts. When you can do that you'll create a desirable frequency shift and the blocks begin to transform. You need to believe you can have it, do it, be it and experience it. What you *think* is secondary to what you *believe* about it.

Your soul's desire may be to reclaim your toned physique and vitality, but if you're holding a belief that your life is 'too busy' to prepare nutritious food, you'll revert to fast food because you've told yourself it's too time consuming to prepare. Our behaviour is the result of our beliefs, thoughts and practices and what we tell ourselves most often. No one can expect to change behaviours around food *without* upgrading beliefs and thoughts around making wellbeing a top priority.

Similarly, if you're saddled with health issues, medication and doctors' appointments, you can still help yourself. Identify what *you* believe about your condition, or your symptoms; if your thoughts are negative or pessimistic they aren't helping. I understand our measure of pain differs from person to person and becoming curious about what beliefs you hold about your health can be challenging to do when you feel unwell. But when you convince yourself that trying to raise the frequency of the area or areas in your body where pain or symptoms are located is worth a go, it can make a difference for the better. You can start over with a fresh approach. Even if you're bed ridden you can use the power of your mind to visualise yourself in radiant health. Call upon the immensely healing power of your soul to guide you forward.

HOW TO LET GO EFFECTIVELY

Forgiveness is the ability to let go of resentments, grievances or hatred. I've observed holding onto resentments can regularly interfere with a person's forward momentum in accomplishing their soul's desire. Forgive everyone. Start with yourself. It is a step-by-step process worth committing to.

The cause of much pain and suffering is caused by the illusion that we're separate from others. We're connected to *everyone*, the energetic links we have with people, places, events and things travel both ways – like the link between your computer and the internet. When one of us feels pain, energetically we all feel the effect of that pain.

No one finds it easy to forgive an aggressor, but forgiving that person heals your soul. You have an energetic bond to them whether you like the sound of that or not, so in order to release yourself from the effect of that bond, you need to release yourself from them. However long you hang onto your resentment will be how long you actively maintain an energetic link between yourself and that person (or group). Forgiving yourself, and them, is the only way to effectively release yourself from being linked to them and any disharmony already caused.

Transforming resentment and releasing energetic links

Start the process of release by focusing your attention and energy on your heart and reach for compassion, forgiveness or acceptance. This approach goes deeper into the realm of unseen causes that are residing in your soul. Doing this will move you into an optimal vibrational atmosphere and align you to your soul's immense power, which is nurturing and healing. Your soul knows how to heal; the ego doesn't (and can't) being unconscious, it doesn't know better and fills your head with negative self-talk making you believe you're right to resist forgiveness, compassion or acceptance. One of the biggest deceptions of the ego is that you'll feel better when you're 'right' and the other person is wrong. The only way to transcend the ego is to keep redirecting your attention and energy back to your heart centre where it will reach your soul.

When we embrace forgiveness we reflect more of our spiritual nature, which is love. The soul knows how to forgive because it's closer to our spirit than our ego.

There are events that occur in our lives that can make no sense to us whatsoever; we can feel betrayal, disappointment and hurt. Dwelling on these feelings whether we are conscious of the emotions that give rise to them or not often extends the pain; it doesn't make sense to continue to harm ourselves in this way when we can bring an end to it. Yet, to forgive effectively we need to hold the intention to let go and keep our attention and energy focused on our heart centre and be prepared to surrender any concept of payback.

Your soul-self has all the nurturing vibrational frequencies you need to heal yourself to re-engage fully in your life – if you allow it. Because your soul-self is the wisest aspect of who you are, it is privy to a much broader perspective of your soul's evolution than you can access through your normal conscious awareness.

Forgiving yourself focuses love inwards and directs healing frequencies into your mind and body. It relaxes the muscles in your face to make you healthier and more attractive. Forgiving yourself is a reminder that you are an Everyday Miracle Maker who has the power and ability to raise the vibrational frequency of any emotion you experience just by choosing to think differently and in a way that is supportive to you. You probably won't forget the situation that happened, but you can radically transform the way you feel about it. It doesn't matter whether that resentment happened a week or a decade ago once you realise that holding resentment against people doesn't make you feel better. Neither does replaying the incident(s) in your head; all it does is trigger all the unsupportive emotions you felt back then; keeping them going is a form of self-harm. It's time to make a commitment to surrender the resentment completely.

When you hold onto grievances you distance and isolate yourself from family, friends and community, which can lead to feeling isolated and lonely.

Forgiveness heals. It's the best medicine to extend to others and yourself. Forgiveness makes the body feel less burdened, lighter and energised. It also helps you reconnect with the parts of yourself that you mentally and energetically split from in order to create that resentment. Forgiveness is necessary to re-experience your wholeness.

Surrender resentments. Just let them go. They're unhealthy to hold onto. Resentments keep you stuck in aspects of your life and stop you moving forward. Revisiting resentments in your mind keeps you living in the past. You have the power to change how you feel immediately. Every time you ditch resentments you make more room for increased wellbeing. Forgiveness allows you to release blaming a person or situation. You have the opportunity to reframe any situation and take back your power over it by reminding yourself you can decide how you want to feel about it.

You might be holding a grievance towards a friend, family member, colleague, or university professor. It could be a situation you felt you had no control over at the time. Make the choice to recognise you're no longer in that situation, event or environment, that your life has people in it now that love and care about you. By releasing resentments you'll have more love available to offer those who love and care about you. *Choose* to energetically neutralise resentments with either forgiveness, compassion or acceptance so they don't affect your relationships going forward. This process takes time, patience and kindness towards yourself. When your soul's desire is to experience a healthier and happier future you'll experience the shift. If you continue to feed unsupportive memories you can become stuck in a toxic loop of mentally replaying the details of any cause of resentment. Instead, open your heart to the power of your soul's love that's waiting to embrace you.

Resentments are like open windows

Picture this, it's a cold night and the fire is roaring, but the house isn't warming up. You don't understand why. You wander through the house looking for the culprit and discover it's an open window. All the warmth the fire has generated is escaping. You close the offending window, the energy of the heat is retained and your home warms up quickly.

Holding and feeding resentments towards others are *your* open windows. Holding onto resentments lowers your state of awareness and your ability to attract desirable people, places, events and things etc.

Your resentments might be directed towards an ex-partner or past lover. In relationship break-ups sometimes we don't want to forgive because we aren't after an apology, we just want a different outcome to the one we are left with. This is why it's more effective to engage your soul in the act of forgiveness – it doesn't get caught up in the personality's needs. The soul sees a bigger picture – wanting to take you away from the stress and energy-drain that holding onto resentment generates.

The more we forgive, the easier it is to do. The power to transform any unsupportive emotion is within you. Engage your soul, and your mind and body can heal faster.

Any time your inner peace is compromised by a person or situation you can restore how you feel by deciding what *meaning* you choose to give it. Love expands and increases the available energy in your body because this is your true spiritual nature.

Conversely, fear contracts and depletes the available energy in your body. Whenever you feel tired, rundown or unhappy check in with yourself to see if you're holding resentments. If you are, choose to set them free. You'll be re-energised, happier and healthier for it.

THE POWER OF SELF-LOVE

We're *all* a work in progress. Self-love is about loving and accepting ourselves entirely as we are *right now*; not holding back on that love for a time we perceive we're more worthy of it. Giving yourself the most love when you're feeling your lowest helps remind yourself that you're worthy of all the goodness the universe has to offer.

Love is the most supportive frequency that connects all creation. It's the greatest unifying power I'm aware of. When we look at the world and intentionally allow the love within our hearts to extend outward we're able to see and experience more beauty around us, which is often hidden by the filters that our judgements create. The ability to love is intrinsic in all of us. Yet life circumstances can lead us to partition our loving feelings. We can withdraw when we feel people don't understand us. Love is like glue; spread it liberally throughout your relationships and you'll feel connected to everyone and everything.

Your ability and capability to love someone else is relative to your ability to love yourself; self-love keeps you aligned to attract opportunities you believe you deserve that will help you accomplish your soul's desire. Self-love isn't about superficial beauty or egoic self-love, it's about honouring your mind, body and soul for the miraculous and powerful creations they are.

When your relationship with yourself is peaceful and loving you take care of what your mind, body and soul needs because you *want* to, not because you have to. The fastest path to healing is caring for your body when it calls out for it; not by ignoring it.

Self-care of your body means respecting it as a vehicle that needs to last a lifetime. Self-care of your mind means speaking kindly to and about yourself, no matter what.

You're in a relationship of self-discovery with your visible (physical body) and invisible (energy body) self every minute of the day – even when you're sleeping. Your body is visible, but your beliefs and thoughts are invisible. You have two bodies, a physical one and its energetic counterpart that you can *learn* to see. Your energy body powers your physical body, not the other way around. As your awareness of your two bodies working together increases so does your ability to observe and reflect on everything you say, do, think and believe. Your ability to keep increasing your level of awareness exists for an important reason; and that is to support you with the evolution of your soul.

Your energy body is constantly receiving subtle impressions through your intuition, but your mind will only pay attention to it *if* you register its importance. This is where discernment is required. Just as you'd spit out bad tasting food, you need to be careful what you allow yourself to ingest energetically. When your focus is on the physical body's needs and not your energy body, its neglect will become evident. When you choose to cultivate and experience positive beliefs, thoughts and emotions, you'll experience more vitality and energy.

Everyday Miracles Makers embrace *both* of their bodies, taking care to keep them both in optimal condition. Your energy body needs your attention and care, just like your physical body.

EVERYDAY MIRACLE MAKER EXAMPLE - ALIGNMENT

Name: Phoebe

Age: 53

Phoebe owned a massage therapist business – a stunning retreat with a team of highly qualified staff working for her. She loved massage, but if her income didn't improve she'd have to close her business and get a job. The thought of giving up her soul's desire made her miserable, but money was running out and her positive outlook was fading.

Phoebe was committed to doing whatever it took (or so she told herself) with vision boards in her bedroom outlining her business with smiling and healthy customers and staff surrounded by symbols of money and abundance. Phoebe went to motivational seminars, spent hours on YouTube at night watching inspirational talks, but most days she felt flat; her business wasn't busy.

I asked Phoebe when she thought of her business what her predominant thoughts were. She said she repeated an affirmation several times a day: 'My business income flows in consistently and clients come to me effortlessly.' But when I asked her if she *believed* that, she shook her head; they were empty affirmations. She felt because there were so many choices for massage in her local community, prices for treatments had become more competitive. It was a classic example of contradictory beliefs and thoughts; her dominant self-talk was stuck in pessimism. She was *telling* herself that she'd have to close her business soon because funds were running out.

I explained to Phoebe that how her body *feels* reflects the low frequency of her thoughts. To maintain her soul's desire she needed to upgrade her beliefs and tell her thoughts to do a U-turn in the opposite direction which will create the frequency shift needed.

When I asked what practical steps she was taking to market her business to new and existing clients I was stunned by the answer. She confessed that she was not only failing to promote her business, but she was complaining to clients that business was tough. She thought sharing her worries with them when they asked about how her business was going was the right thing to do. She was so focused on her problems that she failed to appreciate when her clients came in for a massage they wanted to leave feeling lighter and revitalised, not burdened with the masseuse's problems.

Phoebe recognised that she was out of alignment with her beliefs, thoughts, actions and language and took steps to fix it. This included implementing a simple and cost-effective marketing plan.

Within 12 weeks Pheobe was back in alignment with her soul's desire (her business) and her income was steadily increasing.

Alignment is self-synchronisation.

ALIGNMENT SUMMARY

- When your beliefs, thoughts, actions and language reinforce each other you are aligned and in sync with yourself.

- Resentments are the most significant obstacles to achieving alignment.

- To achieve alignment you need to take full responsibility for all dimensions of your life, including the areas you find unattractive or difficult.

- Direct your mental and emotional energy towards your soul's desire and work to synchronise your beliefs, thoughts, actions and language.

- Achieving alignment and working to maintain it will draw what your soul desires into your reality with greater speed.

- Being misaligned can feel like resistance, a block and being in contradiction with aspects of yourself.

3 ways to practice alignment

- Spend a day noticing the language you're using when talking to people about your soul's desire. U-turn expressions like 'I can't' to 'I can' or 'I don't know how' to 'I know I'll find a way'.

- Put a note in your diary every day to take action towards your soul's desire, whatever that may be – whether it's a new career, socialising more or training to climb Mt Everest.

- Become curious about any negative thoughts and what beliefs in your unconscious might be giving rise to them. When you identify the unsupportive belief work to upgrade it.

*Immerse yourself in creativity,
it can heal your mind, body
and soul.*

Chapter Eleven

KEY 6: CREATIVITY

KEY 6: CREATIVITY

Creativity allows you to express yourself in a way that can be seen, felt, experienced or shared. It's broader than being artistic. Creativity is fuelled by your imagination, but creativity requires output. Designers use their creativity to solve problems, like turning discarded wooden pallets into housing for the homeless, or making inexpensive and fashionable eyeglass frames from discarded plastic bottles. Even capturing your negative thinking down in a journal and turning those thoughts into healthy and helpful ones is creativity at work. It's a valuable action, not just something you think about and never do. Expressing creativity can heal your mind, body and soul.

It can come in many forms:

- Journaling
- Designing a business, product or service
- Planting a vegetable garden
- Painting
- Dancing
- Cooking
- Sewing
- Activities that recharge your mind, body and soul
- Drawing
- Singing

- Giving a talk
- Exercising
- Decorating, renovating or building a home
- Taking photographs
- Participating in projects that help restore the quality of soil, air and water supply
- Researching a vacation and creating an itinerary
- Building something, anything
- Creating characters when playing with your children
- Finding ways to live more sustainably
- Offering support to initiatives that increase awareness and protection of animals and nature
- Adding or removing items from your home or workspace to create your ideal sanctuary

Have you noticed that when you're productively immersed in a creative project you feel less stressed? Keeping your creativity flowing helps you remain agile to opportunities and possibilities. It also helps you remain relaxed, which is the optimal mindset for creative problem solving.

There's a great payoff for being a conscious creator in every area of your life; it keeps you from falling into a rut. Think about an area of your life that you've avoided and choose to direct creative energy towards it. For instance, you may have a successful career, yet socialising feels like hard work so you don't have friends outside work. You *can* invite new experiences into your life – *anytime*. Getting creative in a situation like this is not as difficult as you might think. Think about the possibility of:

- Hosting a dinner or barbeque
- Saying yes to new invitations
- Getting to know the friends of your friends
- Joining a club or a group
- Exploring an interest to meet others who share that interest
- Grabbing a coffee with a neighbour
- Volunteering your time to a cause you value

Everyday you can choose to apply your creativity (or not) to create valuable experiences in your life.

JOURNALING FOR THE MIRACLE-MAKING MINDSET

Journaling is immensely creative because with reflection and insight you can better solve your life challenges. Journaling also captures points in time of your mental and emotional expression and helps you better understand how you can hinder your progress and how your mental and emotional posture at other points in time have supported you in reaching accomplishments. It might surprise you to learn that most people find it easier to recall negative events than positive ones. Studies suggest this may occur because negative events tend to evoke stronger emotional responses from us, making them easier to recall. Unfortunately, this can give us an unbalanced picture of our life. I encourage my clients to keep an Optimism Journal; it's a powerful tool for balancing perception and recording progress. It's also healing in that it can transform confusion into understanding and insight as you write. For this reason I strongly encourage all my clients to begin journaling from day one of coaching with me.

Journaling captures the good stuff that happens in your mind and life. It records what you may be likely to overlook or dismiss, which is why you need to capture content *as* it happens. It also supports you in transforming challenges and building resilience. Flicking back through the pages of your journal will remind you of your resourcefulness, help you hone your self-inquiry questions and develop your intuition. When you revisit your notes on how you've managed and transformed adversity in the past, you'll feel optimistic and know you can do it again.

It's also a place where you can record your everyday miracles, the synchronicities and acts of grace that come your way in pursuing your soul's desire. Remember, you're co-creating with an intelligent higher power that's actively and invisibly working with you to create everyday miracles in your life.

If your intuition is piqued by the mention of journaling, why not start this week? You can journal every day, or a couple of times a week to capture the highlights or the lowlights of the week. Approach the lowlights kindly. When you do, they can be insightful in assisting you to learn more deeply about yourself. *Always* date your entries. You can save your entries in an A4 notebook or your computer. Write to understand yourself better, to gain clarity. I remind my clients, this is an *optimism* journal that stays focused on finding the opportunities and possibilities in what you're noticing. If you find it difficult to keep your self-talk positive, use your journal to capture the negative self-talk, then directly underneath rewrite *exactly* the same sentence or paragraph in a positive and supportive way. It'll help you to understand what you're thinking. It's an effective way to turn around any critical self-talk which comes from the ego.

Your ego is the part of your personality that is unconscious and doesn't know any better, so make it your top priority to educate it. Self-knowledge is priceless. Be your biggest raving fan.

If you're struggling with how to start journaling, try the following prompts to help your writing flow:

- What are you grateful for?
- What do you find challenging?
- What have you noticed has changed in your thinking?
- What have you noticed about your language that has changed?
- What do you overdo or underdo?
- What have you noticed about your beliefs?
- What has changed in your life recently?
- What actions of yours have changed?
- What are you feeling better about?
- What area of your life needs a frequency shift?
- What was the best moment in your day?

→ *Get started journaling by downloading my free Journal Starter Guide, visit everydaymiraclemaker.com*

TURNING CHALLENGES INTO OPPORTUNITIES

When faced with a challenge, activate a creative approach by asking yourself a question: What opportunities lie within this challenge?

Say you had to sell your car because you needed the money to fund your wellness blog. Everyday Miracle Makers understand that giving up the luxury of a car in pursuit of their soul's desire is all part of their transformation journey to convince themselves how committed they are to achieving it. After all, using public transport can result in opportunities to chat with new people. If you naturally strike up a conversation with a passenger, why not tell them about your blog? Who knows, they may be interested in sharing their wellness routines, tips and contacts with you. Not only is that free content for your blog, it's a promotional opportunity too – invite them to subscribe. More subscribers = more advertisers. More advertisers = more income. More income = a new car. And who knows, it could take you into a better apartment or house and further prospects. In *every* challenge there is an opportunity. Invite creativity into your life everyday.

GLOBAL CREATIVITY

Everyday Miracle Makers are naturally predisposed to being innovators because pursuing a soul's desire asks you to:

- Look for opportunities
- Be persistent
- Stay focused on the end game (which helps you remain aligned)
- Understand that *everything* is connected
- Work with a variety of differing relationships, people, places and things to accomplish the desired outcome

Innovators understand it's all about improvement. That's why we're constantly updating our computers, phones and digital devices. We generally accept the product, service, method, approach or idea won't be perfect, but we expect problems to be addressed and fixed to keep improving it.

CEO and bestselling author Ricardo Semler is the epitome of an innovator. At just 21 years of age he took over his father's company and fired 60 per cent of management, believing that a more inclusive organisational structure would increase profits. It did. Turnover went from US$4 million annually to US$211 million. He says that despite having thousands of people working for him they only have two HR staff; his approach is to look after people so that workplace issues don't arise.

Innovation is creative revolution.

Being an innovator doesn't mean perfection. Innovators are focused on delivering a product or service to better serve their customers with a commitment to continuous improvement.

Creativity is never lost only hidden.

EVERYDAY MIRACLE MAKER EXAMPLE – CREATIVITY

Name: Anton

Age: 49

Anton was constantly overlooked for promotion.

He'd worked tirelessly for 15 years for a software company, yet every time he applied for a Director's role which was his soul's desire he was rejected. Each time for a different reason. He became so miserable he took extended leave to regroup and consider his next steps. He considered resigning, but his self-esteem was so low he wasn't sure he'd be able to get another job.

I asked Anton to tell me about a typical workday, from the moment he woke up to the moment he fell asleep.

Everyday was the same. He often ate the same meal for breakfast every day, he ate the same thing for lunch, and at night he went to bed at the same time. Every *single* night. He was living Groundhog Day.

He followed all the rules at work, never questioning or challenging his superiors or his colleagues as he didn't believe he could add any more value to ideas already presented. I asked Anton what creativity meant to him and wasn't surprised when he replied, 'painting, art, drawing…that sort of thing'.

I offered him a broader concept of creativity that he could employ to enhance his work performance and problem-solve. I explained that creativity is a powerful form of energy that we can use to our benefit, *when* we understand how it works. The more creativity you apply in your workday, the more energised you become because you're inviting that energy to work *through* you. Conversely, the more routine and monotony you restrict yourself to, the more restricted your thinking and work becomes.

I asked Anton to find new ways to approach familiar tasks, and to ask himself whether his experience at work could be better. If so, how? This was a radical idea for Anton; he didn't know where to start. He asked: 'How can I apply creativity if I'm not a creative person?' Anton needed a reminder that he is creative. Everyone is.

I encouraged Anton to try to see work challenges and solutions from the perspective of other area managers he worked with. I asked him to mentally place an identified business issue in the centre of a clock face and place solutions at the 3, 6, 9 and 12 positions that might be offered by the managers in other roles. I suggested he adopt their known problem solving approaches. Creativity is also about experimenting; keeping your mind open to looking at alternative or new approaches, all of which can be tested before they're applied to reduce risk and maximise success.

Anton was pleased to discover after using this creative approach to solve a business problem that he could tap into the power of his creativity at any time to solve other business challenges.

When he returned to work Anton made a list of everything in his area of the business he wanted to improve and involved his team and his Director. A fortnight later Anton contacted me with an update, his Director was taking a leave of absence and Anton had been asked to act in his role.

CREATIVITY SUMMARY

- Creativity is fuelled by your imagination, but creativity requires output. It's a valuable action; not something you just think about.

- Creativity is about expressing yourself in a way that can be seen, felt, experienced or shared. It's not limited to being artistic.

- Being a conscious creator in every area of your life keeps you from falling into a rut.

- When faced with a challenge activate creativity to problem-solve, this keeps you relaxed and better mentally positioned to accomplish what you desire.

- Creativity can never be lost only hidden.

3 ways to reboot your creativity

- Jot down a challenge and ask yourself: 'What opportunities lie within this challenge?' Write whatever comes to mind; don't interrupt the stream of your free-flow thinking. Then commit to follow through with at *least* one of those opportunities.

- Look around your home and ask yourself, 'what's one small thing I can do to make my space more inviting and comfortable'? Say it out loud while walking around your house and take action on it. It could be something as simple as hanging a picture that's been resting up against a wall for months.

- Start an Optimism Journal. Write about your day highlighting the great stuff that happened and look for insights and opportunities in any challenges.

"I can manage anything,"
Repeat.

Chapter Twelve

KEY 7: OPTIMISM

KEY 7: OPTIMISM

Optimism is about believing in yourself and your ability to move through adversity trusting that it's all going to work out for you. Optimism helps you interpret what you see in a supportive and helpful way. It allows you to see opportunities and possibilities in your life.

It is easy to be optimistic when pursuing your soul's desire and it's going well, but let's be realistic; at some point you will encounter setbacks, disappointments, rejection and possibly have days when you lose faith in your ability to accomplish what you have your heart set on. Accepting this is likely to happen means you can be prepared and have a strategy in place to support yourself through it and keep moving forward.

Our brains respond more strongly to negative news than positive news; our brains are also programmed with a negative bias for survival reasons, e.g., we need to solve problems to survive. That means we need to work harder to shape our thinking to be optimistic.

The Dalai Lama XIV says in his book *The Art of Happiness*, "Choose to be optimistic, it feels better". He's right. Supportive vibrational frequencies *always* feel better in our bodies and bring an overall increase of energy. When you work at maintaining optimism you can easily apply your creativity to transform any obstacles that appear. Conversely, when you're pessimistic you'll notice challenges are more difficult to solve.

Everyday Miracle Maker Exercise: Improve how you feel

You have the power to change how you feel in *seconds*. Think about a problem you're struggling with. It might be around money for bills, a feeling of discomfort in your body like tightness, or possibly wanting to feel a deeper level of contentment in your life. Choose a current and specific challenge and for the moment tell yourself (believing) how difficult it is to solve this problem and how upsetting this is for you. Allow your feelings to amplify those thoughts. You're likely to be feeling flat and low. Energetically, we will call this the basement.

Now, you're going to frequency shift from the basement to the penthouse. Think about the same issue again, but this time don't think of it as a problem. Think of it as a *personal challenge* that you're keen to transform. Tell yourself that finding a solution will be easy; after all you've solved many challenges in your past. Think about past challenges you found solutions for – at work, home, anywhere. Now remind yourself of the scenario and the details, paying attention to the contrasting feeling in your body to how you felt earlier.

Change is a part of life, you can resist it and get stuck or see it as an opportunity to refocus and keep on moving. If your enthusiasm feels like it's fading, if you find yourself struggling with self-doubt use these practices to move yourself from the basement to the penthouse. When you understand *why* you're feeling the way you are you can immediately create a frequency shift that will quickly change your attitude and bring you back into a positive and supportive place.

Optimism is a *critical* key for the Everyday Miracle Maker to embrace because what you're envisioning and working towards requires you to remain aligned for everyday miracles to transpire. If you allow yourself to dwell on unsupportive self-talk about why something hasn't shown up, you'll generate stress and feel down which can affect your motivation to keep moving forward. Unsupportive thinking doesn't feel good in your body and energetically moves you away from what you are working towards. Negative self-talk manifests as the inner critic. Tune out of it, and instead *choose* to tune in to your inner raving fan. If you think it's not working, keep practising optimism anyway and stay as aligned as you can in your beliefs, thoughts, actions and language and your everyday miracle will be just around the corner.

The 7 self-transformation keys embraced by the Everyday Miracle Maker are not set and forget; they become part of the daily practice of how you live your life.

GROWTH IS UNCOMFORTABLE

We tend to overcompensate our effort, energy and attention in areas we're most comfortable in, and avoid those we aren't. Growth *is* uncomfortable.

Think about the last thing you learned. Was there awkwardness around it? Whether it was learning a language, to drive, to garden or prepping for an interview, the discomfort, whether it was minor or major, was a sign that you weren't feeling self-confident in that area. That's understandable when it is new.

To overcome that awkwardness you need to keep going... push through the discomfort by practising to increase your skill level and knowledge. Before long you'll start to trust in the process and build your confidence in whatever it is you want to get good at.

If you're looking for work or a career change and keep hitting dead ends, stop and look at *how* you're approaching it. If you're only looking for work online you could unconsciously be avoiding physical networking opportunities, and maybe that's the environment where you may meet your next employer.

Supportive and unsupportive habits

Opportunities for growth can be identified in all dimensions of our life if we have the self-awareness to look for them. Everyday Miracle Makers understand the power of habits in how they think and act to help or hinder their progress towards their soul's desire. Everyday Miracle Makers are vigilant to put as much effort into reinforcing their supportive habits as they are in upgrading unsupportive habits to increase their success. Reinforcing supportive habits like waking up early to exercise is helpful because you'll feel better, so it's worth it. Even something as simple as acknowledging a moment by saying "Thank you" to a person who extended you a compliment can become a supportive habit for you – *if* you keep practising this every time you receive a compliment. All too often I hear people ignore or dismiss compliments they receive mid conversation with another person for no sensible reason. Each time you say "Thank you" you are affirming to yourself you are worthy of receiving that compliment and over time that also contributes to increasing your self-esteem, so it makes sense to reinforce it.

Transforming or neutralising an unsupportive habit in the dimension of your life where it is active, for instance, family relationships can release positive energy to flow in *all* your relationships and attract desirable experiences to you. Unsupportive habits are clusters of stagnant energy that rather than flowing through you, occupy space in your energy field and inhibit energy flow to varying degrees, thus the term 'energy block'. These habits are formed from your unsupportive beliefs, thoughts, actions and language that are broadcast from your mind, through your body and into your external world. For instance, you may hold a belief that a relative doesn't support anything you do.

It can play out like this; when you think of that person you become unhappy or angry towards them and may decide to spend less time in their company or perhaps cut them out of your life altogether. Until you are willing to positively transform, or at the least neutralise the belief you are holding about them (and/or yourself) that unsupportive habit will trigger the negative emotions that can make you feel upset, and over time if you allow it to persist it can affect other aspects of your wellbeing. Whether what you believe is justified or not, true or false does not matter.

If the result of your belief or thought doesn't make you feel good or neutral, then the outcome is unsupportive, and maybe it's time to rethink how you are approaching it if you want to experience positive changes in your life. If you keep doing what you've done, you can expect more of the same. Resist making a home for clusters of unsupportive vibrational frequencies to sit in your body's energy field. Show these unsupportive habits the door by upgrading your perception around that person or situation each time it pops up in your thoughts and you'll create the frequency shift that is needed to disrupt that stagnant energy and restore energy flow.

IMAGINATION

Your imagination is one of your most powerful internal resources. It's there to help you develop a mental vision board of your soul's desire and give you insights to solve any challenges (before you attempt physical solutions).

The images that come from your imagination are intelligent energetic broadcasts that are moving through you and the world around you. The more frequently you revisit (mentally visualise) the pictures developed in your imagination, the more power and life you'll give them to activate frequencies necessary to move you closer to experiencing your soul's desire.

Elite athletes understand this concept of mentally rehearsing and use it to run races in their mind; they can see themselves crossing the finish line first and winning the trophy or the gold medal. Their ability can be honed to the point that even though they may be sitting at home with their eyes closed; their muscles and nerves will twitch and fire as if they're *actually* running the race. Your mind obeys your version of reality; if you're immersed in imagining a specific scenario, your body will behave as though it were happening. This knowledge is of benefit to you. When you can visualise achieving your soul's desire in your mind, often, you'll be inspired to act in ways that enable that outcome to be realised.

There's an invisible and a visible component to *everything*. Your soul's desire appears first as a thought in your imagination before it transforms from energy to matter, then to experience.

HEALING WITH IMAGINATION AND INTENTION

Whether your child is troubled, a friend is struggling with a health concern or a parent or grandparent is frustrated and sad about their lack of mobility and independence, in situations like these and others, Everyday Miracle Makers can use their imagination to broadcast high vibrational frequencies of healing intentions towards a person in need or to themselves.

Anytime you're overcome with worry about someone, rather than becoming anxious and stressed choose instead to use your imagination combined with a healing intention directed towards wellbeing. Doing this will benefit you and them because it has to pass through your body first. It's two for one!

Everyday Miracle Maker Exercise: Broadcasting healing frequencies

Just hold an image of that person in your mind with your intention being to see them in a scenario that is the optimal you can imagine for them. For instance, it could be as simple as seeing him or her smiling and looking happy, relaxed and fully engaged in their life. Use your imagination to create as vivid and believable a visualisation as you can. Trigger that optimal state mental picture anytime you recognise you're worried about them. To amplify the healing effect, respond emotionally to the mental picture of them in a state of improved wellbeing. Allow yourself to feel joy by knowing they are more content and peaceful within themselves.

By deliberately broadcasting your intention to a composition of positive mental images designed by your imagination on the screen your mind, and then adding emotion, you are deliberately directing healing towards that person. Anytime you think of this person avoid reverting to seeing them in their current circumstances; instead overwrite that image with your new upgraded visualisation of them. Many clients who have used this technique have shared good news with me of the everyday miracles that occurred for their loved ones.

The same technique can be used for helping pets.

→ *To learn how this technique can be applied in various life situations to help you move towards your soul's desire with less effort and more ease, join the Everyday Miracle Maker online community at everydaymiraclemaker.com.*

*Don't give up. Often all that's
needed is to rest and recharge.*

FIND A MENTOR

When you find yourself too challenged by issues to have clarity around decisions consider finding a mentor. Think about people you admire and ask yourself, what would X believe, think, say and do?

They don't need to be people you know well, but they can be. Perhaps you admire your parents for always maintaining an optimistic outlook despite the circumstances they might have been raised in. It could be a friend in sales who despite being knocked back often, doesn't lose his/her enthusiasm for their product or service. Or it could be a professional mentor that has the focus and attention you desire. Or maybe it's a friend recovering from an illness who has taken courageous steps to restore their wellbeing. Pinpoint what you admire or feel you need and identify this in someone, then borrow their approach to move through and transform the challenges you face. Imagine putting on glasses that enable you to see your challenge through their eyes and take steps they'd take in the same situation. My clients often tell me that they can hear or see me (in their mind) reminding them of the insights they gained during our sessions together. They tap into our connection to help them make better decisions.

We tend to admire the attributes we'd like to have. Learn to emulate. If you get stuck remember that if someone has done it before (and been successful at it) you can emulate his or her road to success. Start researching them. Find out how they transformed their challenges and succeeded at what you want to accomplish.

If no one has done what you want to do, been what you want to be, or had what you want to have, begin by researching the closest thing to it. You're never starting from zero.

Perhaps you've thought about:

- Building your self-esteem
- Buying or building a house
- Attracting love
- Starting a business
- Trying a new approach to release emotional pain
- Reinventing yourself physically
- Changing or stepping up in your career
- Strengthening your relationships with loved ones
- Improving your relationship with your partner
- Learning a language
- Skilfully applying stress management practices
- Ridding your personal life of energy drains
- Travelling
- Returning to study at college or university
- Becoming a professional photographer
- Starting a support group
- Mastering the finance side of your business
- Letting go of resentments
- Becoming a parent
- Allowing love back into your life after a relationship has ended

- Becoming comfortable in your own company
- Learning to save and invest money
- Starting a scholarship or fund
- Learning how to communicate with a loved one that's passed
- Supporting your community with your expertise
- Speaking less, listening more
- Discovering how to relax your point of view from black and white, or
- Learning to give without expectations

ENGAGE THE MIRACLE-MAKING MINDSET

Our self-confidence comes from knowing our strengths. If you know you're good at finances and swimming and your garden rivals those in magazines, then your confidence is likely to be high in those areas. When we feel self-confident, we're more likely to say: 'Yes, I can!' instead of 'No I can't.'

Most people aren't self-confident in all areas of their lives because it's difficult for us to excel at everything. You may not be confident at clothes shopping, but if you don't place value on it, it won't affect your self-confidence.

So what's holding *you* back? Maybe you didn't make the interview short list or were knocked back for a business loan. Perhaps you've been dating unsuccessfully, or maybe you just want a more satisfying life, but you don't know where or how to start. Scenarios like these can affect your self-confidence if you let them.

Everyday Miracle Makers understand there are practical and energetic reasons for why their desires aren't coming to fruition. The practical – they didn't research, plan or action what was required. Or the energetic – they took all the practical steps, but held beliefs, thoughts or spoke about their soul's desire in ways that were contradictory to what they wanted to accomplish.

For instance, say you weren't hired for a job. You may have had the knowledge and experience for the position and *consciously* wanted it, but could have been holding an unconscious belief that you wouldn't get along with a person that worked there. The intensity of that belief can take you out of alignment with that role and you don't get a second interview, despite being highly qualified for it.

When you recognise this is a consequence that can occur, you have a choice to upgrade your beliefs and thoughts immediately – or accept the consequences. Being an Everyday Miracle Maker means practising self-responsibility to create a frequency shift whenever you need it, to broadcast the most supportive vibrational frequencies to draw what you want – to you.

The most powerful form of optimism is self-belief.

EVERYDAY MIRACLE MAKER EXAMPLE – OPTIMISM

Name: Susanna

Age: 57

Susanna's partner had left her to be with someone else. She was devastated. She believed that the relationship was moving towards owning a home together, but out-of-the-blue, her partner moved out.

She'd always known unconsciously her partner wasn't right for her, but said she kept trying to fit a square peg into the round hole. Despite that, she didn't know how to bounce back. She'd become critical of relationships and had lost her buoyant personality. Her soul's desire was to return to the hopeful and positive person she once was.

The first thing she needed to understand was that optimism isn't black or white – people aren't optimistic or pessimistic. Optimism is learnt.

I asked Susanna to think of optimism as a pyramid – it sits at the top; it's the capstone. Each supporting block underneath represents the skills and knowledge she needs to acquire to lead her to practising optimism more easily. Because she had gaps and was missing support blocks in her pyramid her self-structure was wobbly.

I assisted Susanna by showing her how she could transform the resentment she was holding around her ex and others, by avoiding gossip, speaking well of people and situations, and practising gratitude every day.

Every time she converted negative thoughts into positive ones – or at least challenged them to determine whether they were factual – she would raise the frequency of her consciousness. It wasn't long before feelings about herself improved. Six months later she'd met someone she could see a genuine future with and was back to being the confident, hopeful and positive person she used to be.

*Tune out of your inner critic
and tune into your raving fan.*

OPTIMISM SUMMARY

- Optimism is about believing in yourself and your ability to move through adversity because you believe you deserve goodness in your life.

- Optimism helps you interpret what you see in a supportive and helpful way and allows you to see opportunities and possibilities in your life.

- Optimism is being patient and understanding that frequency shifting will produce positive results (even when they're not showing up as fast as you'd like).

- Choosing to be optimistic means you're accessing higher vibrational frequencies of beliefs and thoughts, which supports alignment to achieving your soul's desire.

3 ways to re-ignite your optimism

- If you're feeling upset, stressed, rejected, not good enough or not capable, identify what happened and why you're making it mean something unsupportive. If there is no evidence to support why you're feeling that way, challenge your thinking and U-turn your thoughts.

- Take your mind back to a goal you accomplished in any area of your life. Recall how you successfully transformed your challenges and doubts to keep moving forward. Remind yourself you know how to overcome challenges and accomplish what your mind's set on.

- Commit to practising optimism every day to see opportunities and possibilities all around you. Speak well of people, places, events and things. Focus on what's good in your life and the world. Look for it and you'll find it.

When you can't save it, fix it or change it, stage a comeback after a setback and ride the frequency of new beginnings to amplify the upside.

Chapter Thirteen

KEEP REAFFIRMING YOUR SOUL'S DESIRE

KEEP REAFFIRMING YOUR SOUL'S DESIRE

Sometimes the intensity you have for your soul's desire can wane. Indicators can be:

- Beliefs become judgements.
- A decrease in your body's energy.
- Telling yourself it's too difficult.
- Feeling taken advantage of.
- Mistrusting people's intentions.
- Feeling let down.
- Feeling misled or betrayed.
- Believing results aren't showing up fast enough.

By reaffirming and recommitting to your soul's desire daily you keep it energised, vibrant and alive in your life. One of the ways I do this is through what I call 'Chats With The Universe'. I often practise this on my morning walks and imagine myself having a two-way conversation with a personalised version of infinite intelligence. Some of my conversations sound like this: "Wow, you surprised me, that showed up just when I needed it, thank you." Or, "I'd love your help with this challenge; inspire me with ways to transform it". Or, "Help me be my best at serving others today".

I end by sending a blessing to anyone who I sense needs it, whether they're someone I know personally or someone new that's contacted me directly. This small re-affirming ritual can work for you too. Reaffirming your soul's desire to be an Everyday Miracle Maker is a co-creative process with the form of higher power that you can easily and comfortably relate to.

I find this practice keeps me feeling connected to the greatest source of love and guidance that exists – for all of us.

There's always an opportunity to improve the stories you tell yourself about your life. If you've been living your life through a rear-view mirror, start looking forward. Upgrade the stories of your past so they become supportive stepping-stones for how you got to be the awesome person you are today.

Remember:

- There is no one in the world like you.
- You are immensely powerful. Convince yourself you are.
- No other person *has* or *will* experience life on planet Earth like you.
- Your soul is unique and so are its experiences.
- You have talents and abilities that are still waiting to be revealed to you. Whether you're 18 or 80+, there's a bundle of creative energy waiting to be expressed through you. Your soul's desires need you to be fully engaged in your life to release the energy they contain.

Whether your soul's desire is to feel better in your mind and body, have more energy, earn a degree, move into a dream career, become a professional singer, re-engage in life again after the loss of a loved one, have the family your heart longs for or meet your life partner – believe it's possible.

Remind yourself that you're broadcasting specific vibrational frequencies of your desires into the atmosphere and when you're aligned, it is like sending an energetic arrow straight into a bull's-eye.

Get your energy behind the **7 self-transformation keys** to unlock your miracle-making mindset, and you'll fast-track your way to accomplishing your soul's desire.

THINKING, FEELING AND ENERGY PYRAMID

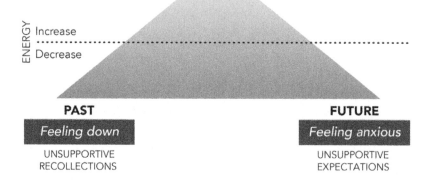

Examples of unsupportive recollections;

- "If I started a savings plan years ago, I'd have greater financial stability"

- "If I hadn't split up with my ex I'd probably be happier than being single"

- "If I had a degree, I'd have a more interesting job"

Examples of unsupportive expectations;

- "I'm never going to make enough money to remain self-employed"

- "I can't see myself travelling overseas with this health condition"

- "What if I say the wrong thing in the interview and I'm not offered the role"

*To protect your results
self-disciplines aren't optional
they're necessary.*

Chapter Fourteen

BTAL ALIGNMENT PROCESS

BTAL ALIGNMENT PROCESS™

These four aspects of yourself can be supportive and help you in accomplishing your Soul's Desire. But they can also be unsupportive and create an imbalance which takes you out of alignment with your Soul's Desire.

Beliefs - What you believe.
Thoughts - What you think - including self-talk.
Actions - What you do.
Language - What you speak, read and write.

BELIEFS → THOUGHTS → ACTIONS → LANGUAGE → SOUL'S DESIRE

STEP 1.

Think about your beliefs, thoughts, actions and language. Do they all positively reinforce each other? If they do, great! You're in alignment with your Soul's Desire.

If you feel they are out of sync, for example your thoughts reinforce your Soul's Desire however your actions are oppositional – it means you're out of alignment.

The most common example of this is when you think one way but act another way.

STEP 2.

To achieve alignment, ask yourself, 'how can I U-turn this aspect of myself and go in the opposite direction?'

If you know your sticking point is aligning your thoughts, then commit to trying new techniques to keep your thinking (and self-talk) moving in one smooth direction towards your Soul's Desire.

STEP 3.

Note in your Optimism Journal how you turned that aspect of yourself around. Include, how it changed how you feel for the better and how it has energised you towards accomplishing your Soul's Desire.

It's also important to note everyday miracles that transpired when you achieved alignment.

STEP 4.

Going forward, whenever you feel any resistance or energy blocks around moving towards you Soul's Desire, it's a sign to check your alignment again – do this by repeating step one.

This process is part of the Accomplishment Formula™

*The universe responds to your
soul's desire by allowing you to
learn it before you earn it.*

Chapter Fifteen

EVERYDAY MIRACLE MAKER FRAMEWORK

History is made by people who refused to give up. Courage grows the more you use it.

EVERYDAY MIRACLE MAKER FRAMEWORK

Learn • Live • Become

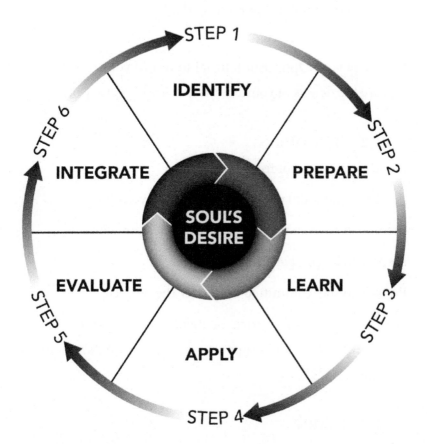

The steps are a cycle that is repeated allowing you to move from learning to becoming an Everyday Miracle Maker to attaining greater mastery.

I developed the Everyday Miracle Maker Framework, BTAL Alignment Process and Thinking, Feeling and Energy Pyramid as support tools.

STEP 1 - IDENTIFY

Allow yourself to accept your Soul's Desire.

Invite it to come through what you value, your interests or a persistent intuitive impulse. It might become known to you through a pain point – something that's currently not working for you.

Note: Use your Optimism Journal to record your progress and capture the details of your everyday miracles as they occur.

STEP 2 - PREPARE

Make a commitment to yourself.

Prepare to take 100 per cent ownership of your life.

Prepare to have an open mind to new ideas and concepts.

Prepare to be completely accountable.

Prepare to stay committed no matter the obstacle.

Get the support of a coach or mentor and become aware of other people who could support you. Support puts you on the fast track.

STEP 3 - LEARN

Fill your mind with new knowledge.

Immerse yourself in the 7 self-transformation keys to unlocking your miracle making mindset. Make them your own and take ownership of their benefits.

STEP 4 - APPLY

Put what you know to work.

When you know better, you do better. Now it's time to apply the 7 self-transformation keys and practices to unlock your everyday miracle-making mindset.

STEP 5 - EVALUATE

Look inward and outward.

Reflect on your experiences, results and accomplishments. Recognise the everyday miracles that have transpired (big or small). Can you identify any new opportunities or possibilities for growth?

STEP 6 - INTEGRATE

Acknowledge what you've done.

Celebrate every win no matter the size. The wisdom you've gained, the effort you've invested and the frequency shifts accomplished to unlock your Everyday Miracle Maker mindset. Pat yourself on the back, it's important and well deserved.

When you say yes to life you become more interested and your journey more interesting.

Chapter Sixteen

YOUR INVITATION TO BECOME AN EVERYDAY MIRACLE MAKER

---

*Step out of your comfort zone,
the universe is waiting
to surprise you.*

YOUR INVITATION TO BECOME AN EVERYDAY MIRACLE MAKER

Ever since I was a young child I had an inner knowing that the energetic world contained information that was valuable for me. I also intuitively knew the physical world contained personal insights, whether it came from people or things around me, overheard conversations or graffiti on bus stops.

Once I realised it was in my best interests to pay attention to the signs around me, I gained a new level of freedom and inspiration; it was like I had a secret life. My ability to freely associate often unrelated things has allowed me to see a much broader view of people and the world we live in.

We're all made from the same stuff. The keys and practices shared in the *Everyday Miracle Maker* are life skills accessible to everyone.

The 7 self-transformation keys provide solutions for you.

- If you're searching for the meaning of life, recognise you're a soul.
- If you've lost touch with your true self, reclaim your authenticity.
- If you're lacking certainty in decision-making, reconnect with your intuition.
- If you're working hard yet positive shifts aren't happening, rectify your alignment.

- If you're too focused on what's missing in your life, revive your gratitude.
- If you're getting more knock-backs than opportunities, reboot your creativity.
- If you're prone to questioning your abilities, re-ignite your optimism.

Recognising you have a soul's desire, or that you're prepared to take steps to reveal it, kick-starts the process of self-transformation. Your mind is conditioned by what you choose to pay attention to and what you're avoiding. Give yourself *every* opportunity to retrain your mind and learn how to look and listen to your life in a fresh way that's supportive to strengthening your positive habits and weakening any negative ones.

You are responsible for developing your level of self-awareness. Consider the possibility that some of what you believe may be your *perception* and not based on facts. Also, give yourself permission to experience real freedom; freedom of thought and positive emotions like love, hope, joy and fun. Recognise these as *accomplishments* and celebrate the feel-good power of them.

The benefits of becoming an everyday miracle maker aren't just personal. As you become more aware that raising your vibration and shifting frequencies to more optimal ones are powerful life skills that bring you what your soul desires, you can more easily envisage how the same principles shared in *Everyday Miracle Maker* can be applied to groups of people, be it your family, community, company or country. We can work to accomplish our personal soul's desires and at the same time join another soul's desire in our collective consciousness so that we can all be healthier, more prosperous, more joyful and experience more love and greater peace.

Becoming an Everyday Miracle Maker is an offering to step into something sacred and much greater than a limited sense of self. If you don't have any physical or emotional challenges you're concerned about, but you're still wondering if there's more to life than what you're seeing, touching and experiencing, the answer is yes. Becoming an Everyday Miracle Maker will open your eyes to a new way of experiencing and interacting with the world around you and within you that allows you to draw even more positive and uplifting experiences into your life. By working with the 7 self-transformation keys daily, you'll learn how to activate the countless everyday miracles that are on standby, waiting to show up in your life.

There's a time for contemplation and there's a time for action. Now might be time to redefine your life for new action. Everyday Miracle-Making is a journey of self-discovery and self-transformation. The way forward is in your hands.

'Turn up your light and together we'll light up the world.'

Infinite blessings

Wisdom is the gift you give yourself when what you've experienced is wholeheartedly understood.

THANK YOU

Writing this book was one of my soul's desires. I'd like to extend huge heartfelt thanks to all my clients, past, present (and future) who've trusted me to guide them through their self-transformational journeys. It's been a blessing being of service to you all and sharing my knowledge of becoming an Everyday Miracle Maker.

To Chey Birch – my cherished long-time friend for the unwavering love and support she provided which made it easier for me to focus on writing whilst balancing other work commitments. I'm eternally grateful for our friendship and blessed by it daily. Chey's own accomplishments are inspirational to me and my gratitude to her is immense.

To Natasha Solley, whose consistent enthusiasm and belief in my message has been like having a cheerleader alongside me. Natasha's support on this project has been unshakable and her love and friendship mean the world to me.

Sam Pease's incredible experience as a bestselling author and television presenter along with her straight-talking and lightning-fast editing skills have kept me on track. Sam's reassurance through the initial writing process helped me enormously.

To Martine Negro – as a mentor she has played a key role in my life. She lectures at Nature Care College (Sydney) and practises acupuncture, Chinese medicine, Thought Field therapy and energetic healing. I was privileged to work at

Nature Care Wholistic and Medical Centre for eight years as a Medical Intuitive beside Martine, Tracy Degeer, Naturopath and Doctor Yvonne (Ruby) Bloomfield. I feel blessed for working with and knowing these intelligent, wise and compassionate women.

I'd like to thank my long-time friend Ann Joel who guided me to make contact with Martine at exactly the right time. Ann continues to inspire me with her energy, enthusiasm and healing work.

To Estelita (Little Star) Dela Cruz Pearce, for her friendship and guidance through out this project. She is a wellness practitioner of many modalities whose own story of healing inspires me. And to my dear friends Sarah Jeffery and Julian Glover whose support and healing gifts have uplifted my spirit throughout the writing.

I first started writing *Everyday Miracle Maker* after meeting Barbara Hoi who helped me develop better strategies to work with dyslexia. Her expertise and passion was immensely helpful to me. I'm grateful to Babs for her awesomeness.

I'd like to thank artist and teacher Kim Roth who has supported and encouraged this project. The generosity of his feedback throughout the creative process was a sacred gift.

I'm grateful to my parents Carmela and Ciro La Pegna who brought me into this life and have given me their most prized possessions; love without end, the value of family and my appreciation for good Italian food!

My grandmother Nina Miragliotta for her support and love and also for teaching me resilience, which she has abundantly demonstrated throughout my life.

My three siblings; Emilie, Nina and Luis and brother-in-law Maurice for their never-ending love and support. They're uniquely precious to me and each occupies a special place in my heart.

I'm fortunate to be the Aunty of four darlings; Sara, Chiara, Alessia and Alexander who became my first students (unknowingly) and are still as enthusiastic about Aunty Silvana's educational chats as they were when they were little people. I love and adore the four of them; thinking of them *anytime* always makes me smile.

Special thanks to my spirited niece Sara whose expertise in a range of creative disciplines meant she received more calls from me that she probably anticipated or wanted on this project. Thank you darling and appreciation to Damiano for supporting all you do.

To Jane Penberthy, for our friendship and her expertise and enthusiasm that helped me maintain momentum. I'm so grateful.

And to friend Tina Croker for her unwavering support, insights and assistance when it was coming down to the wire. My heartfelt gratitude.

To Mal Carnegie, whose expertise I recalled from a serendipitous conversation. His contribution allowed me to meet my deadline. And for that I'm greatly appreciative.

To Julie-Ann Harper (and her amazing team), who unknowingly to both of us was drawn into working with me by a synchronicity that reconnected our friendship and allowed me to benefit from her publishing expertise and guidance – thank you, thank you, thank you!

To all my extended family and friends, I'm enormously grateful for your encouragement and support of my work and referring me to your friends, family and colleagues – bless you.

To my many teachers of spiritual development and coaching around the world who've helped me deepen my knowledge, expertise and understanding, I send you my love and profound gratitude.

I'd like to acknowledge the infinite consciousness that I purposefully co-create with daily to experience my everyday miracles. It's because of its consistent and powerful presence in my life that I feel compelled to share what I know so that it may also help you.

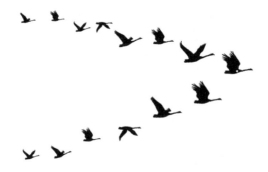

TO CONTINUE THE JOURNEY

For further information, to book coaching sessions or purchase products visit everydaymiraclemaker.com

> Free resources

> Personal coaching

> Group coaching

> Programmes

> Events

> Speaking

> Sacred Light Aromatherapeutic Mist

> Join me on social media

> Join the Everyday Miracle Maker community for updates, really helpful tips and to share your journey and everyday miracles.